Restructuring
Health Care

J. Philip Lathrop

Booz•Allen Health Care Inc.

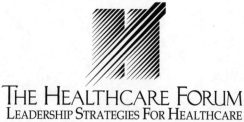

THE HEALTHCARE FORUM
LEADERSHIP STRATEGIES FOR HEALTHCARE
•LEADERSHIP CENTER PUBLICATION SERIES•

Restructuring

Health Care

The

Patient-Focused

Paradigm

Jossey-Bass Publishers · San Francisco

Substantial discounts on bulk quantities of Jossey-Bass books
are available to corporations, professional associations, and other
organizations. For details and discount information, contact the
special sales department at Jossey-Bass Inc., Publishers.
(415) 433-1740; Fax (415) 433-0499.

For sales outside the United States, contact Maxwell Macmillan
International Publishing Group, 866 Third Avenue, New York,
New York 10022.

Manufactured in the United States of America

The paper used in this book is acid-free and meets the
State of California requirements for recycled paper
(50 percent recycled waste, including 10 percent
10% POST
CONSUMER postconsumer waste), which are the strictest guidelines
W A S T E for recycled paper currently in use in the United States.

The ink in this book is either soy- or vegetable-based and during the
printing process emits fewer than half the volatile organic compounds
(VOCs) emitted by petroleum-based ink.

Library of Congress Cataloging-in-Publication Data

Lathrop, J. Philip.
    Restructuring health care : the patient-focused paradigm / J.
Philip Lathrop.
        p.   cm. — (The Jossey-Bass health series)
    Includes bibliographical references and index.
    ISBN 1-55542-594-1
    1. Health services administration.   2. Medical personnel and
patient.   3. Medical care—Philosophy.   4. Patient advocacy.
I. Title.   II. Series.
    RA971.L32   1993
    362.1'068—dc20   93-29550
                                                                          CIP

FIRST EDITION
HB Printing   10 9 8 7 6 5 4 3 2 1   Code 9396

The Jossey-Bass

Health Series

Contents

Contents

6. Patient Aggregation: From Nursing Units
    to Patient Care Centers   110

7. Initial Deployment Decisions   134

8. Enablers for Change   158

9. Does It Work?   182

    Epilogue: The Patient-Focused Enterprise   205

    Recommended Readings   211

    Index   215

Foreword

Several years ago, The Healthcare Forum developed a compelling organizational vision: **to create healthier communities by engaging leaders in building new visions and models of care.** This vision has driven our work ever since. It has served as a screen through which we have scanned the universe of leadership theory and practice for transformational strategies, methodologies, competencies, and values that would help leaders create these new models of care. Into our view came patient-focused health care delivery.

Why is patient-focused care transformational? Because it shifts the structure of health care operations from a fragmented, overly specialized, bureaucratic, delay-prone model to a new paradigm focusing on the patient's perspective and fundamental needs. Through cross-training staff, it minimizes labor costs while increasing the continuity and quality of care for the patient. Bureaucracy and waiting time are significantly reduced. Patients feel better when cared for by a core interdisciplinary health team.

The community receives better value from its health care delivery organizations.

Emanating from operations research, patient-focused health care delivery has a conceptual connection to two other major areas of The Healthcare Forum's work—systems thinking and continuous quality improvement. Results of pioneering work by Booz·Allen Health Care and others have been introduced to the health care field through The Healthcare Forum's executive conferences, *The Healthcare Forum Journal,* and our Operational Restructuring Compendium, which profiles nineteen pioneering hospitals that are utilizing patient-focused models of care delivery.

Now comes a book to further document this seminal work and show how it can be applied. *Restructuring Health Care* is insightful, well-written, and easy to understand if you work in or with hospitals and clinics. We think you may have an "aha" experience as we did when we first learned about the patient-focused approach to health care delivery.

Restructuring Health Care is endorsed by our Healthcare Forum Leadership Center. We are developing a number of action-oriented leadership publications and learning tools. Over the next several years, we plan to extend our endorsement to selected books whose ideas and authors support our vision. To find out more about our programs, publications and Leadership Center, please call 415/421-8810.

Our best wishes to all of you who become advocates and practitioners of patient-focused care. Your organization, patients, and community will benefit from this transformation. Let us know about your journey.

San Francisco   Kathryn E. Johnson
July 1993   President and CEO
                                                   The Healthcare Forum

Preface

The efforts of hospitals to reduce costs and improve service hit a brick wall in the mid 1970s. The late 1960s and early 1970s had been hectic years of extending the capacity of the system to meet the demands of patients newly enfranchised by Medicare and Medicaid. In the subsequent decades, the opportunity and compulsion to improve performance were clearly present, but evidence of improvement would be hard to document—even after making allowances for the absence of price competition and the rapid expansion of technology, both of which have contributed to the increased cost of health care. The litany of mitigating factors is well known: greater intensity of care, increasing capital costs for facilities and technology, more regulation, defensive medical practice, and so forth. None of these, however, adequately explains the rapid and continuing rise in personnel costs or the underlying problem with service levels.

What has made poor performance such an intractable problem in health care institutions? The culprit is the same that has stymied significant progress in virtually every other human endeavor: blindness to the underlying assumptions; in other words, the limitations of our current way of thinking. Recognizing that we ourselves—not immutable laws of nature—impose the limits is a difficult but transforming step in the restructuring process. In current business shorthand, this is called a paradigm shift. For those at the forefront of such change, it is more akin to an out-of-body experience, and often requires a whole new vocabulary and map for the foreign and sometimes frightening landscape that is revealed.

Purpose

The purpose of *Restructuring Health Care* is to take the reader on a guided journey into this new world and to provide a totally new set of optics for viewing health care institutions today. Despite the pain of reentry into the old world after this visit to the new, it is hoped that the reader will be moved to *do* something. This is the frightening part of the journey—leaving behind (or better yet, challenging) the old world and its entrenched ways.

Patient-focused care has gained great currency in the health care field in recent years, largely as a result of seminars, articles, and discussion about the efforts of the early implementers. Like most ideas that spread rapidly, however, its meaning has broadened without any concurrent deepening of understanding. In fact, it has become in some ways a catchall for any number of initiatives—from minor efforts at cross-training to full operational restructuring. Although the book does not attempt to divide such efforts into orthodoxy and heresy, it does for the first time gather between two covers both the theoretical and the practical underpinnings of the paradigm shift. No series of brief articles or visit to a restructured hospital can reveal the genesis of the the concepts or the theory that supports their development. This book is intended to fill that void in a clear and readable way.

Audience

Patient-focused care, patient-focused restructuring, and *patient-focused hospital* have become nearly interchangeable terms. At one level, the overlapping usage is fine. As the ideas evolve, however, the terminology risks becoming a limiting factor. In its broadest sense, the paradigm shift is about *all* health care operations and activities—not just hospitals and not just the inpatient side of hospital operations.

Considering the evolution of the concepts to date, the logical audience for *Restructuring Health Care* is hospital leadership (including the board, top management, and departmental directors). But the problems addressed by patient-focused care are no less present in ambulatory care settings, long-term care facilities, home health agencies, and even doctors' offices and clinics. Furthermore, as health care achieves greater vertical integration of services within settings, the boundaries within the system will become more blurred. Patient-focused care should be considered a set of tools and ideas to be applied to health care operations in the broadest possible sense. Their origins in the inpatient arena should not limit their application in other settings. Given this perspective, the potential audience for this book becomes "the field": doctors, nurses, and other professionals who deliver or manage care in all settings. Because of their role in preparing tomorrow's managers and practitioners, educators should also become conversant with patient-focused care and seek to extend its concepts into their curricula and beyond.

Although this book is unlikely to enter general circulation, laypeople (that is, patients) might find it interesting as well, if only because it shows why their experiences with the health care system are so often confusing and unsatisfying. Putting the book into patients' hands might provide additional pressure for change. Laypeople are hereby invited to ignore the bits of jargon and read on. They are likely to hear their own stories being told.

Finally, managers and operations specialists in other businesses will find many analogues in health care to their own problems. The methodology used to create the concepts of patient-focused care is equally useful in other situations—especially service businesses that struggle with highly variable demand and an ever-present temptation to centralize and standardize.

Overview of the Contents

Restructuring Health Care presents both the why and the what of patient-focused care. It also includes examples of what has happened at various hospitals. A separate volume would be needed merely to begin an exposition of possible approaches to implementation. I therefore leave issues of process and detailed design to subsequent research on the subject.

The introductory chapter argues for a renewed emphasis in health care on operations management—breaking away from the field's mimicry of industrial organization models and management at a distance. Chapter One seeks to shake the reader loose from the notion that everything is all right or just needs some fine tuning. The task of turning the world upside down should not be taken lightly. The first glimmer of a diagnosis appears in Chapter Two, which offers a formal explanation of how we got where we are today and what scope of change will be needed. The third chapter carries the diagnosis further and gives the malady a name—compartmentalization.

Chapter Four shifts the focus to the demand side of the operations equation, arguing that if we are to fix the supply-side problems identified in the first three chapters, we must start by understanding our customers' needs—how and when they occur, and how our traditional responses fall short. The "treatment plan," if you will, starts in Chapter Five, where I outline the structure of the new paradigm and discuss its implications not only for care at the bedside but also for management of the enterprise.

Chapters Six, Seven, and Eight begin the discussion of new ways of viewing how we group patients (including outpatients), location of services, and selected approaches to patient-focused care, respectively. The final chapter presents the results of implementation at some of the pioneering institutions.

The Epilogue deals with the next few years of patient-focused care and also reflects on its place in the broader restructuring that we are likely to see over the next decade, in light of the changes in the health care system being contemplated at the federal level.

Acknowledgments

Though I am the author of the book, I am by no means the sole source of the ideas and results it presents. The book represents the collective knowledge and vision of a number of talented, courageous executives who wanted to make a real difference in the care of patients in hospitals and other health care institutions.

I have had the privilege of being involved from the earliest stages of the patient-focused hospital's development. My role for the past two years or so has been to proselytize to the industry about patient-focused care. It is a task that I have assumed with enthusiasm and a sense of mission. If frequent flyer miles are any measure, I have by now spoken to a sizable proportion of the nation's hospital managers and executives. The adoption of patient-focused care has not been especially rapid, but its momentum of late has increased substantially. That is a tribute to the message, not the messenger.

The ideas in this book might not have been formulated without the clients who honored us with their trust and shared their problems and insights. The concepts would not have their power had it not been for the partners and staff members of Booz·Allen Health Care who worked long hours wrestling with problems that had seemed intractable for decades. Acceptance of patient-focused care would not be growing without the efforts and experiences of more than thirty hospitals in the United States, Britain, and Australia that have bravely implemented what so many thought was foolishness, if not outright heresy.

The book is dedicated to all those who have toiled or will toil on behalf of patient-focused care. It is a noble venture, whose benefits accrue to the people we serve. There will be crises ahead, but the journey will be worth the hardships, and the results will be worthy of our goal.

I wrote several versions of these acknowledgments, identifying individual executives at client organizations and my partners and former partners at Booz·Allen. However, it became obvious that the staff members who did the real work and the client executives whom we served are too numerous to mention, and I might inadvertently leave out key contributors. You know who you are and should take great pride in your achievements. To the clients who granted permission for some of their data and experiences to be shared, I extend a special measure of thanks.

Chicago, Illinois   J. Philip Lathrop
July 1993

The Author

J. Philip Lathrop is vice president in the Chicago office of Booz·Allen Health Care. Since joining the firm in 1976, he has led a broad range of consulting engagements for top management of many of the leading hospitals, systems, health maintenance organizations (HMOs), proprietary chains, and professional associations in the United States. Since 1988, he has devoted nearly all his time to working with clients on the development and implementation of patient-focused care. Mr. Lathrop is also a frequent speaker and writer on the subject and a member of the faculty of the Governance Institute.

For three years before joining Booz·Allen, Lathrop was assistant administrator at Talmadge Memorial Hospital in Augusta, Georgia. He received both his A.B. degree (1971) in biological sciences and his M.B.A. degree (1973) in hospital administration from the University of Chicago.

When not working or traveling, Lathrop enjoys spending time with his wife, Lynda, and his stepdaughter, Rebecca, at their retreat in Maine, doing crossword puzzles and driving race cars.

Restructuring
Health Care

Introduction

This book is about the development of a new paradigm for health care operations—rediscovering the fundamental nature of the services provided in an institutional environment and pursuing those insights to their operational conclusions. The modern hospital has no operational equivalent in any other human endeavor. It is a twenty-four-hour hotel with no effective reservations system or useful demand forecasts. The variety of potential services to a particular patient is virtually incalculable. The most commonly cited and compared benchmark (full-time positions per occupied bed) is typically five or more, translating into the equivalent of one employee being at the side of every patient every minute of the day (including allowances for weekends, holidays, vacations, and leave).

    Not since the zenith of assembly-line manufacturing have we seen such fragmentation and specialization of a work force. In American automobile factories of recent decades, one could find employees whose sole jobs were to attach chrome trim to the passenger side of vehicles coming down the line. The hospital equivalent today finds employees who only draw blood (from veins, but not arteries), people who admit inpatients but not outpatients, staff who file insurance claims but cannot process cash payments, housekeepers qualified to clean tile but not carpet, and on and on. Hospitals mimicked industrial organization models but failed to respond to the operating challenges and imperatives inherent in a high-technology service business.

It should surprise and perhaps shock us to be in a field that spends almost nothing on research and development in its core concern—the day-to-day operation of a complex, labor-intensive service business. When surveys ask about "hospital problems," executives seem to trot out all the usual suspects: Medicare and Medicaid reimbursement, the uninsured, the AIDS crisis, difficult doctors, unreasonable patient expectations, and so forth. The only characteristic shared by all these issues is that there is precious little that any one institution can do about them. They are policy-level black holes, consuming vast amounts of energy but emitting no light. What would we think if hotel general managers attended several conferences a year to wring their hands about the effect on their business of the price of gasoline or rising air fares? We would probably tell them to stay home and make sure the front desk is efficient, the rooms are clean, and room service arrives on time. We would also expect them to reinvest some of their profits in research into how to do their business better. We should expect no less of ourselves—reemphasizing the importance of customer service and backing it up with investments of time and money.

This journey into the future of hospital operations is a work in progress. The effort is now about five years old and began with a group of pioneering clients who knew there had to be a better way. They were tired of business as usual and unhappy with the choices that the traditional world offered: essentially short-term, evaporating savings purchased at the cost of low morale and static or deteriorating service levels. The paradigm was broken, incapable of solving a staggering number of real-world problems. The challenge was—and remains—to find a new system with which we can liberate ourselves from rising costs and declining performance.

As in the early stages of any paradigm shift, there is ample room for disbelief and a great desire for proven results. Unfortunately, at this stage, it is difficult to provide any such guarantees. There is a growing list of problems we can solve and demonstrate using the new paradigm. Step changes in service performance are being documented and sustained over time. Turnaround times for routine procedures are being reduced by two-thirds. Improvements in patient satisfaction easily eclipse those previously thought possible. Physicians are finding that they can spend more time with patients without increasing their time on the units. Extrapolated savings continue to meet predicted levels. No one who embarked on the journey is turning back; they are just getting farther and farther ahead of those waiting to make sure it is safe to begin. Nevertheless, definitive answers to all questions, a completely restructured hospital, and audited documentation of savings are still to come. At this point, pioneers with faith in the new order continue to live in the risky and murky middle ground that lies between today and tomorrow. Their reward is the challenge and excitement of leading the way to a better future.

You will find no academic footnotes or learned bibliographies on your journey through the ideas in this book. It is not an arcane bit of research accessible only to the initiated. Though rooted solidly in the fundamentals of business, this work is not rocket science. It requires only common sense, an open mind, and the willingness to ask new questions and pursue the answers wherever they lead.

1

What's
the Big
Problem?

Hospitals have no shortage of internal and external measures of their operating performance. Full-time-equivalent (FTE) positions per occupied bed, housekeeping hours per thousand square feet, relative value units (RVUs) per medical technologist, nursing hours per patient day, and so forth can be tracked internally over time and compared to regional and national data bases for hospitals of similar size and mission. Administrators and department heads learn to talk in the shorthand of such reports and are not above presenting them to their boards when the comparison is favorable ("Ain't we *great*") or even when the comparison is less than favorable ("Ain't we *different*"). But these measures are also limiting. In a sense, they measure only ends, not means. Process and structure are left out of the statistics, creating the need, in fact, to explain away variances. The numbers also imply that we can manage what we measure. Sometimes this is true, as in the case of housekeeping productivity; sometimes it is not altogether true, as in the case of RVUs per technologist (since neither management nor the technologist has any significant control over laboratory demand plus or minus 5 to 10 percent).

A fresh look provides some stunning and disturbing characteristics of the modern hospital. Much of the early work on the patient-focused hospital was led by operations specialists, not hospital managers and traditional health care consultants. Their backgrounds were in the manufacturing, banking, and retail industries. They had never seen the inside of a hospital professionally, but they brought in-depth skills in operational analysis. They were a bit awed and confused at first but soon uncovered facts that, while amusing, were also deeply troubling.

The Clerk Paradox

Most hospital executives would scan Table 1.1 with equanimity. Familiar figures displayed in a familiar format, showing total employees by category for a hospital with an average daily census of about 450 patients. A quick mental calculation of FTEs per occupied bed yields a comfortable number (about 5.23, unadjusted for part-time employees and outpatient volume). The numbers and the calculations are so familiar, however, they have nearly lost their meaning.

The data point in the table that merits a fresh look is the number of clerks and secretaries: 455. In and of itself it is just a number, about 20 percent of the total staff. But think again. The clerks and secretaries outnumber the inpatients! Exaggerating to make a point, we could reorganize the hospital and give all inpa-

Table 1.1. Employees by Job Category.

Category	Employees
Managers and supervisors	147
Administrative professionals	100
Clerical support	455
Nurses and technicians	1,196
Laborers	424
Total	2,322

tients their very own clerk on day shift (a sort of latter-day Radar O'Reilly). The clerk would stay with the patient and write down everything that happens—nursing notes, doctors' orders, vital signs, and even charges. The clerks could produce handwritten, real-time bills. The hospital could discard its billing computer.

Although this is not really a serious suggestion, the example serves to illustrate the surprising culmination of years and years of incremental change using the same basic operating assumptions. It also gives an initial glimpse into the fact that writing things down has become the biggest single activity in our hospitals. But there are other mysteries to be uncovered.

A Radical Management Approach

There is a management equivalent to the "clerk paradox." If one counts up all the managers and senior staff in a typical 300-bed hospital, one will find at least eighty of them at or above the department-head level. If you doubt this figure, simply count the noses at the next monthly department heads' meeting. Hospitals everywhere have adopted the same basic organizational approach: functional alignment. In other words, we define and compartmentalize a given activity or function (for example, dietary, admitting, and pharmacy). We then appoint a department head, usually someone who for his or her entire career has performed the function to be managed. It is almost unheard of for someone in a hospital to be managed by an individual with a different functional or professional background. This incestuousness breaks down somewhat at the vice president–assistant administrator level. Here we have generic executives managing clusters of semirelated functions (ancillary services, support services, administrative services, and the like). It is all very neatly and reflexively logical.

But wait. What has this produced? Is there a different way to marshal these eighty or so managers? The answer is yes. We could relieve them of their current functional responsibilities and redeploy them. There are enough of them to allow us to have a

CEO for every three or four patients. Instead of running Central Supply, for example, that manager could be appointed President and Chief Executive Officer of Rooms 322, 323, and 324—accountable for managing or arranging for all the resources the patients in those beds require. And these would be high-prestige jobs because we could assign two or three secretaries to each of these new-breed CEOs.

In one sense, this is not a serious suggestion, any more than the Radar O'Reilly concept was. In another sense, it raises troubling questions about the fundamental ways that we organize ourselves to manage the modern hospital. Implicitly, if not intentionally, we have come to place a higher value on functional background and depth than on general management skills in our selection of leaders. Although this practice is understandable and reasonable, its pervasiveness at virtually all levels of the organization results in an extraordinary number of compartments, multiple layers of management, and limited spans of control.

A typical hospital of three hundred or so beds will have upwards of one hundred activity centers—some with departmental status, others with section status within departments. On the surface, this situation is neither good nor bad. But when we examine it in more detail, the prevalence of narrow spans of control becomes apparent. Figure 1.1 displays the sizes (in FTEs) of the activity centers and departments in a 500-bed hospital. When we look at the distribution of activity centers by size, we find that 62 percent have fewer than ten FTEs. This pattern repeats itself in hospital after hospital, reflecting the similarity in operating structure across the nation, and for that matter the entire world. The question for our purposes here is whether this basic organizing principle is effective in managing costs and service levels for patients.

Terrible Customer Service

Quality is a major issue for hospitals today, both within the field and in the more general public arena. Unfortunately, for the vast

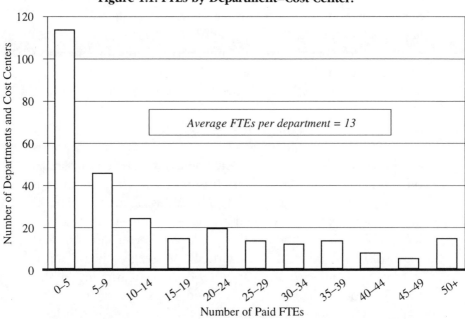

Figure 1.1. FTEs by Department–Cost Center.

majority of hospitals, the current emphasis on clinical outcomes is probably misguided. The major problems of quality revolve around customer service and process quality rather than the question of whether the vast majority of patients go home with excellent clinical and scientific outcomes. This is not to say that such issues are inappropriate or that we should ignore them. The problem is that the tools we use are by and large post hoc and statistical—treating the care process as a black box. Since the process is so complex and involves so many different people, such gross measures may be the best we can do. By all means, let us quantify overall outcomes and pursue the problems we find, but there is much more we can do in addressing the broader and deeper meanings of quality.

The technical and scientific armamentarium of modern medicine is one of the triumphs of our field. We can now diagnose and cure conditions that could not even be accurately described just twenty years ago. A triumph of nearly equal proportion is that we have managed to convince the customers of the modern hospital (patients and physicians) that what we provide is good service. It is unusual to find a hospital whose patients do not report being satisfied at least 80 or 90 percent of the time. By and large, internal surveys of physicians offer similar results. In addition, administrators can honestly state that they are not inundated with complaints from patients and their families.

Yet just as our assumptions about operating structure have blinded us to the excessive clerical work and management layers in our organizations, we need to look afresh at defining the issues of customer service. Traditional patient surveys are not the way to measure customer satisfaction, any more than looking at FTEs per occupied bed should be our primary yardstick in assessing operational effectiveness and efficiency. Hospitals, like most other service businesses, ask the wrong questions. They ask questions whose answers can be dealt with within the existing paradigm. For example, think about your last stay in a hotel. In all likelihood, you had the opportunity to complete a brief customer service questionnaire. Somewhere on that form was a question like "How was the service at the Front Desk?" (poor, fair, good, excellent). We are so used to this process that we do not even think about whether the question is sensible or if the answers will be truly useful. It is a question posed in a form that management can deal with, not one designed to elicit untidy information. It is a question that begs its own answer and assures that nothing significant will change based on the responses. Think about it. The hotel customer does not need a Front Desk. The hotel customer requires an empty, clean room with the right type and number of beds, designated either smoking or nonsmoking, and the proper key to fit the lock. The customer probably also needs to know that he or she will be billed the proper amount and have adequate documentation for reimbursement. The client may also need assistance with luggage and directions to the room. Nowhere on this list of real customer needs is a Front Desk. It is simply the structural approach of the hotel to providing these essential services.

The hospital equivalent of this example is to ask "How was the service in the admitting department?" (poor, fair, good, excellent). Again, our customers (in this case, patients) do not really need an admitting department. In response to this question, a patient might muse, "Gee, it was great—all sixty minutes of it!" If we are serious about customer service, we need to ask much better questions. How long did you wait? How many irrelevant questions did we seem to ask? What should we have already known but asked anyway? How long were you at the hospital before any care was actually delivered? How many questions were repeated after you arrived in your room? How many forms did you sign? How many of those forms did you understand? We probably know the answers to many of these questions already but feel that we are structurally unable and philosophically unwilling to pursue the root causes of the problems they point to.

The following sections highlight several operational parameters that we take for granted today but that should cause us to reconsider our sometimes complacent attitudes toward customer service.

Excessive Turnaround Times

The average hospital requires about four hours to process and deliver a routine service—an initial drug order, a lab test, an X ray exam. Physicians might see turnaround time as short as two hours if they are lucky, six hours if they are not so lucky. When we try to diagnose this problem, it is difficult to find the culprit. Those on the nursing staff will say that they transcribe the order within ten or fifteen minutes; the couriers can demonstrate that from the time they get the order until it is delivered to the pharmacy is only fifteen minutes or so; the pharmacy has studies showing that from the time it is aware of the order until the time it is ready for pickup is only twenty minutes on average; and so on. Each piece of the process seems to be well executed, but in the final analysis the service is just too slow. Most frustratingly, even if we could improve the performance of one of the subprocesses, there is little hope that the impact on total delivered time would be significant or noticeable.

Our customers have subtle ways of telling us that the system is broken or at best not always responsive to their needs. If we look at high-volume tests in the hematology and chemistry sections of the laboratory, we will usually find that in excess of 50 percent of all such tests for inpatients are ordered "stat" or some other equivalent. Does this mean that in over one-half of the cases lives are hanging in the balance? Of course not. It is more likely to mean one (or more) of the following things:

- The physician ordered the test a few minutes after the deadline for that service cycle (for example, all tests ordered by 7:00 A.M. will be drawn and run, and results will be posted on the chart by 11:00 A.M.). If it is 7:15 and you want the results that morning, you are forced by the system to order it stat.
- The physician, from personal or rumored experience, does not trust the laboratory to meet its promised delivery schedule.
- The physician will be leaving the hospital for the day in an hour or two and does not want to go through the trouble of calling in to get the results for that patient's tests.
- The faculty attending physician will be making rounds in two hours, and the second-year resident realizes that he or she forgot to order a test that the faculty member always requests.

This list could be produced for almost any department in the hospital. In each case, we should read these maneuvers not as selfish or dishonest but as the result of a rigid, one-size-fits-all approach that is failing to meet our customers' needs.

Continuity of Care Crisis

Perhaps the single most troubling result of today's operating structure is the number of different employees who interact with

**Table 1.2. Number of Staff Members Interacting
with Patient (Four-Day Stay).**

Category	Average Number of Contacts
Nursing	27
Dietary	10
Ancillary services	6
Central transport	5
Environmental services	3
Other support	2
Total	53

a typical patient during a three- or four-day hospital stay. To accomplish all the tasks involved in a four-day colectomy stay involves fifty-three different staff members (not counting doctors), as shown in Table 1.2.

These numbers may seem an exaggeration, but they are quite realistic. Think about the nearly endless stream of people who parade in and out of a patient's room—those passing out menus, those passing out trays, those collecting trays, those picking up linens, housekeepers, nurses and their assistants, clerks, transporters, respiratory-care staff members, those starting intravenous devices, and so forth, often with different staff each day and on each shift. It is no exaggeration to say that continuity of care is a contradiction in terms. Further, since the work is so compartmentalized, no one can be held accountable for the bulk of patient care; in essence, no one "owns" the patient.

This situation leads directly to a common complaint of patients: the "I'll get someone to do that for you" syndrome. We all know how this goes. A patient asks the nurse for some ice chips for his water pitcher. The nurse says, "I'll get someone to do that for you." This is all too frequently followed by the "You mean they haven't done it yet?" syndrome when the patient rings the call button fifteen minutes later and repeats the original request to the nurse. In many cases, however, the patient's request can be handled by the original contact person in less time than it takes to track down the "appropriate" employee, transmit the service request, and make sure the task is properly performed.

There is another situation that happens far more often than

it should and that is a direct outgrowth of the lack of continuity of care. All patients (the conscious ones, anyway) are likely to experience the following situation at least once during their stay. A nurse looks into the room and asks, "Has respiratory care been in to see you yet this morning?" This is a perfectly understandable shortcut for the nurse to take. The alternative for getting this information is to go to the nursing station, find the chart (if it is there), find the right entries for respiratory therapy, and decipher the handwriting to see if today's treatment has been given. It is much easier simply to ask the patient. The problem, however, is that after this happens a couple of times the patient starts to wonder (with some justification), Doesn't anyone know what's going on around here?

Our difficulty in coordinating the actions of fifty or more people in the care of a single patient is only one problem created by compartmentalization. As we will see later, the high cost of all these limited-task doers is also a by-product of the structure.

Priority Given to Institutional Convenience

About the last thing hospitals take into account in arranging the sequence and timing of services during a patient's stay is that person's desires and preferences. Our attitude seems to be that it is better that six patients should wait than one machine be idle. All too often, the day begins something like this: "Good morning, Ms. Jones, it's 5:30. Please fill this cup in the bathroom. When you come out, we're going to stick a needle in your arm. Then we're going to throw breakfast in front of you and ask you to eat it quickly because you have to go to X ray and we need to clean your room. Good morning." This summary may exaggerate to make a point, but it contains more truth than it should. At the end of this book, we will return to this scenario in more detail to illustrate a broad range of problems with the current operating structure and to suggest means for making fundamental change.

Of course, it is not only our inpatients who are put through cumbersome processes. The problems of the current operating structure can be understood more succinctly by looking at a set of common outpatient procedures. Consider the following True-Life Adventure involving an outpatient referred to the hospital for a chest X ray, a complete blood count (CBC) and an electrocardiogram (EKG). This is a major ordeal likely to involve nearly a half day of walking and waiting.

The Odyssey

This odyssey begins at 9:30 A.M. in the hospital parking lot. Having found a place to park, the brave outpatient enters the building with doctor's orders in hand—get a chest X ray, a CBC, and an EKG. Thank goodness it's nothing complicated, thinks Helen Jones. I should be back at the office in time for my lunch meeting.

An efficient and attractive information desk looms before her ("Visa and Master Card Accepted" —a good omen). She is efficiently directed to the nearby Registration Waiting Room. Her heart sinks as she sees the crowd and signs in at the bottom of a long list. She thinks, Oh well, at least they've got lots of clerks. Perhaps the wait won't be too long.

Thirty-five minutes (and several year-old People *magazines) later, her name is called. The list of inquiries begins: name; address; social security number; home and business phone; husband's name and occupation and employer's address; number of children; next of kin not residing at the same address; insurance coverage . . . . "Wait! I'm going to pay in full and handle the claim myself," a frustrated Ms. Jones blurts out.*

"Sorry, but we need that information anyway," the clerk says sympathetically.

The questions continue—plan identification number; referring doctor's name, address, and phone number; allergies; medications; previous admissions; major illnesses; religious preference; and on and on. Finally, the lengthy form is presented to Ms. Jones for signature. Fifteen more minutes down the drain. But at least something could actually happen now.

"Take this down the hall to the outpatient cashier," the clerk says, smiling.

"Can't I just pay you?" our heroine asks.

"Sorry, all payments and insurance arrangements must be handled by the cashier."

The chairs in the cashier's area are a bad sign; another wait is certain. Given the almost total lack of privacy, she inadvertently learns that some patients are going through tortuous Medicare Paperwork Hell to pay for an X ray and others are making arrangements to bill insurance for outpatient surgery. Isn't there an express lane for direct payment on three items or fewer? she wonders. Alas, no. When finally served by a cashier (ten minutes later), she is sure the worst is over. Now she can get her tests done and go home.

"Thank you very much," the clerk says; "take these receipts and follow the yellow stripe on the floor to radiology."

Great. Now *things are happening.*

Gee, the Yellow Brick Road was shorter than this! she moans to herself. After a few minutes, though, she arrives at radiology. As she steps to the registration desk (no line!) she notices a patients' lounge to her right. Oh, no. Lounges and waiting rooms are built for a purpose, she thinks. There wouldn't be one here if I weren't about to need it. Her lunch meeting today is becoming little more than a dim hope. After presenting her paperwork and receipt, she is given a form on a clipboard. The form seems eerily familiar (name, address, referring doctor, child-bearing history and status, previous X ray work at the hospital, and so forth). Her patience wearing thin, she approaches the radiology receptionist.

"Why do you want to know if I've had X rays here before?" she asks.

"So we can pull them from the file room for comparison," answers the cheery clerk.

"But it was six years ago—for a sprained ankle!"

The clerk now realizes he has a "problem patient" on his hands. "Just fill out the form, please," he adds with an icy note of finality. Ms. Jones returns to the lounge to wait. She calls her office to alert them to the probability that she will have to reschedule her lunch meeting. It is 11:00 A.M.

After a fifteen-minute wait, she is summoned by the technologist. A quick change from her blouse into a hospital smock, stand up to the wall, lift the chin, hold the breath, click, whir, and it is over. About three minutes total, by her reckoning. She changes into her blouse and goes back to the receptionist, nearly regaining her optimism and faith in humanity. The radiology receptionist (a new one, covering the lunch hour) directs Ms. Jones to the outpatient blood-drawing station. "Just follow the red stripe on the floor."

The walk to the drawing station at first seems like a movie running backwards—very familiar scenery—and then, voilá, the outpatient registration area looms ahead. But the red line runs right through it and continues for another fifty yards! Making some vague connection in her mind, she wonders, Do you spell Bataan with two A's or three? Ms. Jones is learning the system fast, though. She knows she is in the right place when she sees The Waiting Room. The paperwork here is pretty simple, and the wait is only ten minutes. The phlebotomist is very efficient and finds a vein and draws a tubeful of blood in about a minute. Once you get past the paperwork and waiting, these people do a good job, Ms. Jones begrudgingly admits to herself.

The home stretch is in sight, she now allows herself to think. The laboratory receptionist directs her to the blue stripe on the floor, at the end of which she will find the Heart Station. She realizes this is where her EKG will take place.

This walk is much shorter than the previous two, but she still wonders how many heart patients may have died en route. Trying to forget how hungry she is, Ms. Jones presents herself. Again, the paperwork is nominal (but also seems unnecessary and redundant), and is followed by the standard fifteen-minute wait. The magazines here are especially old—presumably moved here after spending at least a year in the main registration lounge. Lying on the bed waiting for the technician, she examines the EKG machine beside her. The color-coded instructions are on the lid! Why don't they let me do this myself? she wonders, only half-kiddingly. The minutes click by on the wall clock until the techni-

cian finally appears, places the electrodes, whirs the machine for
thirty seconds, and tells her to get dressed and go.

It is nearly 1:00 P.M. Despite her hunger, she decides to
avoid the cafeteria, escape the hospital, find her car, pay $4 for
parking, and go buy stamps at the post office, where she is certain
that she will receive better service.

This is hardly a user-friendly process. One of our Catholic
hospital clients refers to this as the Stations of the Cross approach
to outpatient services: we seem to ask our patients to reflect and
do penance at each point in process. It does not have to be this
way, however. To experience the first glimmers of what fundamental restructuring is all about (and the quantum leaps in service that can be accomplished), let us revisit the hospital with
Ms. Jones after some radical changes have been made.

The Return

"Everything looks fine, but I'd like to get some standard diagnos-
tics done for you," Dr. Smith tells Helen Jones.

"Oh, please, don't send me back to that hospital for tests.
Last year it took three-and-a-half hours to get three simple proce-
dures done!" she pleads.

"I'm sorry about that. I know it was cumbersome, but I
hear they've made some changes. In fact, they now guarantee
that if you arrive for simple tests between 10:00 and 2:00, they'll
be done in less than an hour—or you don't pay. Why not give
them a try?" Dr. Smith suggests.

"Well, all right, but I don't know how that's possible. I think
I spent nearly an hour just walking from place to place last year,"
sighs Helen.

Approaching the hospital, she notices some reassuring
changes. Signs direct her to an outpatient drive-up entrance with
a staffed valet parking stand. Thinking back to the previous year,
she immediately suspects a gimmick to raise parking rates and
extract a tip. She is pleasantly surprised to read the sign on the

*stand—"Complimentary, No Tipping." Well, this is more like it.
I don't pay to park at the mall. Why shouldn't the hospital be the
same? she thinks. The valet gives her a claim check and pulls away
in her car.*

*"Hello, may I help you?" she is immediately asked as she
approaches the outpatient reception desk. "Yes, please. My name
is Helen Jones, and my doctor referred me for a chest X ray, a
blood test, and an EKG."*

*"Fine. That shouldn't take long at all. It's 10:30 now; you'll
be on your way by 11:30 at the latest. Please take a seat, and
someone will come get you shortly," advises the receptionist.*

*Oh great, thinks Helen. Now they've got people to lead me
by the hand as I wander all over this place. Big improvement.
I'm glad I brought some crackers to see me through lunch. At
least the tests will be free this time.*

*Ten minutes later, a well-dressed young woman ap-
proaches. "Ms. Jones? My name is Mary Johnson, and I'll be handling your visit today. If you'll follow me, we'll have you out of
here in no time."*

*Helen is escorted into a small, well-appointed office with
a desk, chairs, computer screen, nicely decorated cot, and an EKG
machine on a cart. "Please make yourself comfortable," Mary
suggests. "I just have a few basic questions before we begin."*

*Right, Helen thinks cynically. Good thing I brought my Filo-
fax this time.*

*"I see you're here for a chest film, CBC, and EKG," Mary
begins, "I'll just need your name, address, and phone number."
Helen quickly provides the information, feeling more relaxed
about this experience.*

*"Since you're getting an X ray, I also need to know if you're
pregnant and if you've had X rays here before," says Mary.*

*Oh, here we go again! Helen thinks to herself. "No, I'm not
pregnant, but I did have a chest X ray here last year. I suppose
that will make me wait while you track it down."*

*"No need to inconvenience you. If the doctor wants to see
last year's film, we'll pull it. But you can be on your way without*

worrying about that," Mary assures her. "Okay, one more thing. How do you want to handle the charges?"

"Visa, I'm afraid. I'll have to go to the cashier I suppose," sighs Helen, remembering last year's experience.

"Absolutely not, I can handle that right here," Mary says as she begins filling out a charge slip. In no time at all, she takes an impression of Helen's card and hands her the receipt along with a crisp printout of services received, prices, date, hospital provider number, and other items Helen knows the insurance company always needs.

"Now, if you'll slip out of your blouse and put on this smock, we can get started," Mary says as she goes out the door to allow Helen some privacy. "I'll be back in a minute or two."

Helen's cynicism makes her wonder if the hospital's new system now requires her to walk the halls in an institutional smock. She also begins to speculate about how many more employees she will have to deal with as the process unfolds. She is both surprised and delighted to see Mary reappear as promised.

"Let's do the EKG first," Mary suggests as she pats the cot.

As Helen lies down, she asks Mary, "When will the technician get here?"

"She's here, and she's me," Mary answers. "I've been trained to do everything you need today. You see, I'm a registered radiology technologist, but I've also been trained to register patients, handle payments, draw blood and other samples, and perform EKGs. It wasn't that hard and, besides, we have specialists available if I need help or something unusual comes up. We think it's a better way to serve our patients with fairly simple needs than to send them all over the hospital."

"Well, you've got my vote," Helen volunteers. "I felt like a pin-ball in slow motion the last time I was here." As she removes the EKG leads, Mary invites Helen to have a seat so she can draw the blood sample.

As Mary draws the blood (on the first try), she explains to Helen, "We also figured out that if we could get people to come in after our morning rush of scheduled patients and ambulatory surgery arrivals, we could really serve them quickly, especially if staff members could be trained to meet a variety of their needs. That's why we can give a one-hour service guarantee for most straightforward procedures and tests."

"You're doing great so far, but I don't see an X ray machine in here. Do I have to go to radiology?" Helen asks, her skepticism still showing.

"Don't worry. It's just around the corner, and you won't go through any public areas to get there. We have two machines in this area, and while you were changing I was making sure one would be available for us now. They were both busy when I checked; that's why we did the EKG and drew the blood first. I'm sure one will be free now," Mary tells her. "Just leave your things here. I'll lock the door on our way out."

Good to her word, an X ray room is empty. The procedure takes two to three minutes. As Mary escorts Helen back to the office and unlocks the door, she says, "You can change now. While you're doing that, I'll take your blood sample down the hall and be right back."

Helen is just picking up her purse as she hears Mary's knock on the door. "Come in," she says. "This was too easy, Mary. Are you sure we're done?"

"All done. I'll walk you back to the reception area. I'm going there for my next patient," Mary tells her.

As she hands the valet her claim check, Helen notices the unopened crackers in her purse. "Time for a real lunch today; it's only 11:15."

The transformation described in the two stories does not happen overnight and is especially complex for inpatients. But the potential benefits for customer service and hospital costs make it incumbent on us to imagine the future in more detail and to take steps to achieve a new vision of our operations.

The Worst of Both Worlds

Poor service in hospitals might possibly make sense if, say, twenty years ago a group of experts had sat around a table planning the hospital of the future and said, "Yes, we know we will give bad service, but think of the money we will save for our patients!" But poor service is not cost effective. We now have the worst of both worlds—high (and increasing) costs, combined with poor service. The cost side is perhaps the more troubling dimension since over the past two decades so much effort (internal and external) has been devoted to attempts to control costs. Beginning with Medicare's routine cost caps and continuing with such efforts as utilization controls, productivity monitoring systems, investments in computer systems, and even across-the-board cuts, nothing has had any serious, positive effect on the overall rate of cost increases for hospital services.

Every day, in hospitals across the country, CEOs and other senior managers sit at their desks and try to improve cost and service performance. They pull the "levers" that they have been taught to pull to change the organization. But these levers do not seem to be connected to anything. Significant change continues to elude us. We reach out to new techniques like total quality management (TQM) or continuous quality improvement (CQI), throw resources at them, and hope for the best.

We now know the missing ingredient in today's operational dilemma. It is an understanding of the impact of structure on cost and service performance. Without this understanding, we are fated to continue to repeat the "doom loop" of recent years—superficial change, leading to insignificant and temporary reductions in costs, followed by deterioration of service levels and further erosion of employee morale. If, however, we can uncover the true sources of performance, we will be able to shape a new vision of hospital operations. This vision will reinvigorate our organizations and unleash the power of techniques (for instance, TQM) that have been hamstrung by our existing structural paradigm. The vision will also liberate the creativity of managers and employees once they see that the system can be meaningfully changed and that they can have a personal impact on the quality of care and service in our institutions.

2

The Nature of

Structural Change

Restructuring is a term heard round the world these days. The popular and business press are full of company announcements of restructuring. In everyday parlance, it usually translates into layoffs. In some cases, this cynicism is probably justified. More often, however, the changes described by restructuring are in fact quite different and more profound than layoffs. It implies a fundamental shift in the way a company does its business, or at least some portion of its business. Perhaps the most accessible example of a true restructuring is General Motors's recent creation of its Saturn division. This was no mere downsizing, assembly-line acceleration, or factory closure. It was a complete rethinking of the way that American cars are designed, developed, assembled, distributed, marketed, and sold. It required a major investment of time and capital, driven by the realization that the old paradigm just could not solve the problems of quality, cost, and global competitiveness.

On a smaller scale, we read about insurance companies

restructuring their claims-processing activities. They are moving away from an assembly-line approach where one clerk logs in the claim, another checks it for accuracy and completeness, the next enters it into the policyholder's file and computes the amount actually to be paid, and finally another clerk processes a check request—all separate from the complaints and adjudication requests that may come in after the check is received by the claimant. Restructuring in the insurance industry generally takes the form of small teams of multiskilled employees being responsible for the claim from the time it is received until the policyholder is satisfied. Anyone who has dealt with the bureaucracy of an insurance company would have little hesitation if asked which approach they would find more responsive. The extra benefit to the insurance company is that the restructured approach is less costly and results in lower employee turnover rates.

Restructuring often appears to be obvious and easy in retrospect, perhaps like the claims-processing example just given. Unfortunately, it is seldom that straightforward. Our traditions and personal experiences blind us to the problems at hand; in other words, we seldom recognize that there really is a problem. Hospitals are especially guilty in this regard because of their complexity, the number of specialists who are relied upon for the last word in their areas of expertise, and the very seriousness of health care itself. Managers and care givers go to their own national and regional meetings and are reassured that since everyone else does things the same way and has the same problems, everything must be okay—or at least "that's just the way things are."

But we can do better. If we honestly and objectively analyze the operating structures of hospitals using some basic tools from operations research in other industries, we can begin to see the problems in a new light. This chapter focuses on some of the theoretical underpinnings of a structural approach to performance improvement in hospitals.

The Concept of "Value Added"

It is both obvious and worthy of emphasis that if we are going to improve cost and service performance in hospitals, we must begin by looking at how we use our employees—how many there are, what kinds, what we ask them to do, how we organize them, and how in reality they spend their time and the institution's resources. At the end of the day, it is people who provide service, and it is they who account for the bulk of hospital expenditures. Figure 2.1 shows a typical breakdown of hospital expenses.

A reporter once asked Willie Sutton, the famous bank robber during the Depression, "Willie, why do you rob banks?" "'Cause that's where the money is," he replied with brilliant simplicity. Although this is admittedly a crude formulation of a key operating principle, it is nonetheless useful in looking at hospitals or other businesses. If we are interested in improving cost performance in hospitals, we need to begin with personnel-related

Figure 2.1. Hospital Cost Structure.

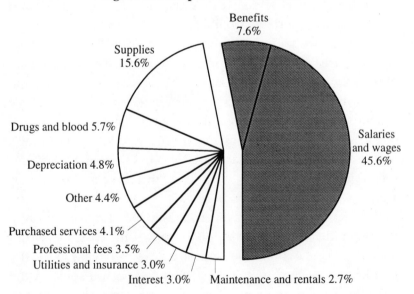

Benefits 7.6%

Supplies 15.6%

Drugs and blood 5.7%

Depreciation 4.8%

Other 4.4%

Purchased services 4.1%

Professional fees 3.5%

Utilities and insurance 3.0%

Interest 3.0%   Maintenance and rentals 2.7%

Salaries and wages 45.6%

costs. These usually account for 50 to 60 percent of all expenditures. As a simple matter of directing our energies most effectively, it is easy to see that even a modest improvement in personnel-related costs will dwarf much larger percentage improvements in any other cost category. This situation, combined with the fact that personnel are also generally responsible for service quality, makes the direction of our initial inquiries obvious.

The concept of *value added* goes to the heart of an enterprise—essentially dividing the inputs of production into two categories, raw materials and value-added activities. For example, silicon is a raw material for the production of microprocessors; engineering know-how, design, fabrication and assembly, and distribution are value-added activities. Adding value is not therefore a social concept or even a judgment as to whether a given activity produces anything worthy of its cost, although in the economic long run it must.

For hospitals, the value added is the sum of all personnel-related expenses, and the two expressions will be used interchangeably throughout this book. All the other cost components of a hospital's activities will be viewed essentially as raw materials. For instance, unexposed X ray film is a raw material. The value added in producing a radiology consultation is the sum of all labor costs (direct and indirect) necessary to schedule the procedure, document its steps, transport the patient, perform the procedure, develop the film, review the image, type the report, file the film, and bill for the procedure.

But the value added is simply a category of cost, not the answer to any profound question. It helps us understand the nature of our businesses at a macro level. When we analyze the components of a hospital's value-added structure later in this chapter, we will find some surprising facts. Before that analysis can be made meaningful, however, we need to make one more observation about the overall cost structure of the hospital and present a framework for thinking about costs in a new way.

The Idea That Hospitals Are Capital-Intensive

The literature of hospital management and the conversations of hospital executives are liberally sprinkled with the notion (or at least the suspicion) that we are in a capital-intensive business. The annual and long-range budgeting cycles are dominated by issues surrounding the upgrading of facilities and the acquisition of new technology, not to mention the debt that is required to make all this a reality. But take another look at Figure 2.1. Total capital costs (interest plus depreciation and amortization) are less than 10 percent of overall hospital expenditures. Nationally, these items amount to about 9 percent of total cost. So where is the capital intensity?

We need to recalibrate our scale to understand the situation. A capital-intensive activity is a $300 million petroleum cracking plant with a modest staff of operators, engineers, and security personnel. Between raw materials (oil) and capital costs (depreciation and interest), we may be looking at 80 to 90 percent of total cost. This is hardly the situation in a hospital.

The perception of hospitals that they are capital-intensive springs from a different source. Hospitals have historically been cash poor, a situation that seems just like being capital-intensive. When we do not have the cash to purchase all the new gadgets we want, it is an easy leap to the conclusion that we are in a capital-intensive business. But this is an important mistake. Hospitals are labor-intensive enterprises; the belief to the contrary can lead us down the wrong path when we make long-term decisions about the capital-to-labor trade-off.

We should be able to look at the capital-labor equation and make some simple calculations about the implied trade-offs. For example, if we assume a given capital asset has a useful life of, say, eight years, we discover that the expenditure can be justified if the equipment in question saves just one-eighth of its total cost in annual operating expense. Put another way, if we can save $10,000 per year in operating costs, we can spend roughly $80,000 in capital and be economically indifferent.

Hospitals seldom think in these terms or place any great credence in the ability of technology actually to reduce annual operating expenses. We have been disappointed too many times to be fooled by this naive type of analysis. It seems that every time we invest in new technology—despite its promises—we seem to end up with more operating expenses (usually people) than when we started. For example, that powerful new laboratory computer system that was supposed to save twenty FTEs of nurses and clerks in fact resulted in no staff reductions, but rather the addition of two computer specialists to keep it functioning effectively. So much for the capital-to-labor trade-off in hospitals.

The good news, however, is that we can indeed gain operating leverage by judicious investments in technology. Some of these, as we will see, are not necessarily investments in the latest technology, and some will be investments that the traditional world would view as duplicative. But their cost effectiveness is real and their impact on customer service significant.

A New Framework for Cost Performance

Not all costs are created equal. This fact of life became obvious when manufacturers tried to improve their cost performance. What was needed was a framework that recognized the differences between costs and the different strategies to which each might or might not be susceptible. As a result, operations strategists devised a conceptual model for thinking about costs: the cost performance hierarchy (shown in Table 2.1).

The basis of the hierarchy is the realization that there are different costs, incurred for different reasons, over different periods of time, about which we can do different things operationally. At the highest level of the hierarchy are *inherent* costs. These are the ones we incur by deciding *what* we will do in our business—essentially, costs determined by our very decision to be in a certain activity. For a hospital, this would mean deciding, for example, to be a 300-bed institution in an urban area of the Northeast, offering maternity care, psychiatry, general medicine

Table 2.1. Operations Performance Hierarchy.

Category	Composition
Inherent Level: "<u>What</u> is done?	Census and admission rates Variability of demand (external) Intensity of care required/severity of illness Quality of care objectives Service offerings Location
Structural Level: "<u>How</u> is it done?"	Organization structure Management processes Operating policies and systems Capacity management Physical size and layout Equipment deployment Skill mix
Execution Level: "<u>How well</u> is it done?"	Productivity levels Work pace Skill level

and surgery, open-heart surgery, and a large emergency room and outpatient clinics. We will incur certain costs as a result. We need a building of a certain size and minimal equipment. We must heat, cool, light, and insure the facility. We will be subject to the vagaries of the market in which we find ourselves—population size, structure, and growth rates; incidence rates of various diseases; local Medicaid reimbursement features; land prices; and so forth. Inherent costs are sometimes referred to as strategic costs since having any effect on them really requires a change in the overall strategy or location of the business itself.

The next level, the *structural* one, is the most interesting for our purposes. This is the level in the framework where we decide *how* we will do what it is we have decided to do at the inherent level. Here we make literally thousands of implicit and explicit decisions about structuring the work to be done. For hospitals, this process means answering many questions. Will we have twenty- or thirty-bed units? Will we use primary nursing or team nursing? Will phlebotomy be a centralized function, or will it be performed on the units? How many departments will we have? How many vice presidents are needed in the structure? Hospitals tend to leave most of the truly interesting questions on the table—assuming that the approach everyone else uses is the right one. This tendency is magnified because of the way hospitals interpret the role of the Joint Commission on Accreditation of Healthcare Organizations (JCAHO). The JCAHO sets standards in a way that appears to codify the status quo. In fact, the index to the standards is a list of departments in the typical hospital. Thus, virtually every hospital adopts the implied operating structure. The standards are actually open to a number of structural solutions, as the recent experience of several restructured hospitals would support. The JCAHO does not have to be a major obstacle to rethinking hospital operations and may in fact be a source of support and encouragement.

Finally, we get to the *execution* level. Here we address questions of *how well* we perform, given our strategy and structure. This is the classic productivity level of the framework, focusing on questions such as is the work pace too fast or too slow, is the skill mix too rich or too lean, and do we pay too much or too little in the marketplace for skills? This area has received the bulk of management attention over the years. Investments in management engineering staffs and productivity monitoring systems are the most common inputs. Even when done scientifically, the outcomes are usually across-the-board staff reductions. This is sometimes called the "work harder and faster" approach to operations improvement. There are a number of problems with focusing management efforts at this level, each of which is discussed in the following sections.

The Perversity of Productivity

Productivity measurement is all well and good—as long as we measure the right things. Unfortunately, in hospitals, we find ourselves forced to measure activity at the department or section level. These activities are not necessarily items the organization wants to maximize or optimize. For example, in today's world, we would commend the department head who succeeds in increasing the number of patients moved per transporter and thereby decreases the unit cost of each patient move. But wait, did we really intend to set up a measurement system that would be successful when it was able to move more patients through the hospital more often? Of course not. By measuring units of "intermediate" products or services, we invite abuses that arise from simple manipulation of the system. This problem is also apparent in areas like the laboratory, where we almost unquestioningly accept engineered standards of relative value units (RVUs) whether they match the reality of our lab's methods, staffing, or demand patterns. Productivity measurements also imply that what is being measured can actually be managed. Within broad limits, this is not always the case. Most departments in the hospital benefit from increased census when their productivity numbers are reviewed. In most cases, they no more deserve praise for these "improvements" than they deserve criticism when the census declines the following month and their productivity numbers go to hell.

Productivity standards can also lull us into complacency; they can lead us to believe not only that what they measure are the right things but also that the way we do those things (the very underpinning of the "standards") are the right ways to do them. The following True-Life Adventure illustrates the folly of both these assumptions.

"Productivity Is Up. I Need More Staff."

"Great news, Ms. Henderson. Productivity is up 20 percent in records assembly," Jack Wilson tells his boss. Jack runs medical records at the hospital, and Ms. Henderson is the chief financial officer.

"That's really good to hear—a welcome relief from the usual bad news. I'm glad something is improving around here. The CEO is all over the senior staff to cut FTEs, and I was beginning to think I had run out of options. Jack, you're a real life saver," Ms. Henderson gushes thankfully.

"Yes ... well, it's not that simple," Jack stammers as he watches Ms. Henderson sink down in her chair.

"It never is, I suppose. Fill me in step by step." Ms. Henderson suspects what she is about to hear would be hilarious if it were not true.

"Well, you remember why we set up records assembly in the first place?" Jack begins. "When we did the accounts-receivable audit, we found out that many unbilled accounts were sitting in medical records waiting for all the loose sheets to arrive and to be put in the right charts. You know, lab work and X rays from the last day or two of each stay. We decided that the improvement in cash flow justified hiring people who would spend all their time filing loose sheets and completing records so the accounts could be billed faster."

"Were we right?" asks Ms. Henderson.

"Hard to say. Billing-cycle time is down maybe a day or two, but the reduction in carrying costs of that is probably only $50,000 to $75,000. With benefits, the filing clerks probably cost us $80,000 to $100,000," Jack estimates. "But even so, we'd be drowning in loose sheets without these people."

"Okay. Go ahead," Ms. Henderson prompts.

"Last fiscal year, each assembly clerk filed 180 loose sheets per day—a hospitalwide total of over a quarter million sheets per year, if you're curious. During the last six months, they're handling nearly 220 sheets per day. That's where the 20 percent productivity improvement number comes from," Jack continues.

"That sounds good to me. Why isn't that the happy end of the story?" wonders Ms. Henderson aloud.

"Because the total flow of loose sheets now exceeds 240 per clerk per day." If nothing else, Jack has got the numbers on this stuff.

"Why is that? Census is virtually unchanged—a bit down, if anything," counters Ms. Henderson.

"Oh, all the usual reasons—acuity is higher, whatever that means; there is more defensive medical practice; and so forth. I think it's equally likely that nursing units just send the charts

down sooner, since even modest completion is no longer their concern. That translates into more loose sheets coming to medical records," Jack opines. "Normally, if the backlog were temporary, I'd simply suggest some overtime to eliminate it and get us back on an even keel. But that won't fix this problem, since the increased rate of loose sheets has held steady for the last quarter."

"So what's the answer, Jack?" asks Ms. Henderson, holding her head in her hands.

"Well, the productivity factors indicate we need two more FTEs, but I'll do my best to get by with just one. Maybe we can find ways to work a bit faster," says Jack almost apologetically.

"All right. All right. I can't argue with the facts. I'll make the request at tomorrow's senior staff meeting and do my best to justify it. You can help by getting me some fancy overhead charts to show the increased work load and productivity," she tells Jack.

"Thank you. I wish this weren't necessary," Jack adds as he heads for the door.

"Just one more thing, Jack," Ms. Henderson calls out. "Don't let any of your people increase their productivity by 40 percent. We can't afford it."

We will return to this example in a later chapter and restudy the issue of medical records productivity from a structural point of view. We will show what can happen when we begin to measure the right things and open ourselves to a broader definition of the problem.

One final example of the problems of productivity measurement is necessary. It shows the ultimate perversion of the sometimes tedious mechanisms used to track the productivity of our staff. As part of an exercise to educate top management about how their organizations actually function, we often ask them to write shadow stories. These are composed after a senior executive follows one employee through an entire shift to see how his or her time is spent. One particularly enlightening shadow story came from observing a respiratory therapy supervisor on the evening shift at a 200-bed hospital. The supervisor was a "player-coach"—that is, not only responsible for supervision of three staff members but also expected to perform her share of the procedures that were ordered. During the first forty-five minutes of the shift, the supervisor went to her office and sat in front of her computer. While she did this, the other three therapists sat and waited. And what was the supervisor doing at the computer? She was scheduling and equally distributing the procedures to be performed on her shift, not because of the complexity of the scheduling but to be certain that each staff member had the same number of RVUs. The productivity system was being used to reduce the number of employees, beginning with those who had the fewest RVUs, so the supervisor was going through this tedium to protect her staff. In simpler times, the four of them would have simply divided up the patients based on their conditions and locations and gone about their business. Today, nearly three man-hours are wasted on the shift to provide grist for the productivity mill. No wonder productivity is a problem.

The Dominance of Structural Cost Decisions

Most hospital cost performance parameters are driven by structural cost decisions. In fact, by the time we have made our inherent- and structural-level cost decisions, we have probably accounted for 75 to 80 percent of total cost. What is left to be determined at the execution level may be as little as 20 percent. It is little wonder that our efforts over the past twenty years have not produced significant, sustainable improvements; there just is not much opportunity in this area. Furthermore, any results we do achieve tend to be short-lived because we are not changing what or the way work is being done.

We can illustrate the dominance of structural cost decisions by looking at pharmacy services. Let us assume we decide to structure our pharmacy services like those of every other hospital of, say, two hundred beds or more. It will have most, if not all, of the following features:

- A large central pharmacy, open twenty-four hours a day
- A retail and/or outpatient outlet
- Two or more satellite pharmacies in high-use areas (for example, the intensive care unit or coronary care unit)
- Floor pharmacists for several other areas of the hospital
- A unit-dose system
- An intravenous admixture area
- A turn-key computer system
- A full-time director
- Two assistant or associate directors
- Staff for scheduling, training, and other support work

By the time we make these structural cost decisions, we have really predetermined most of our personnel-related costs in the pharmacy. How fast an individual pharmacist counts pills or types labels just does not matter very much. Once we staff the various locations and work areas required by the structure, the productivity of a pharmacist is already bounded by fairly narrow limits. Unfortunately, most productivity measures revolve around line items per pharmacist, despite the fact that he or she has little control over demand and almost no control over the structure of the operation that limits potential.

Phlebotomy services offer an even clearer example of the importance of structural cost decisions. Let us say that we have decided (like most hospitals) to have a central pool of phlebotomists dispatched from the laboratory to draw blood samples from inpatients. The alternative is to have unit-based staff members draw blood samples as part of their other care-related duties. But if we decide to centralize the function, it is hard to improve the productivity dimension. Let us say that we encourage the phlebotomists to run from room to room as they perform their rounds. First, any noticeable impact on laboratory turnaround time is unlikely since sample collection is only a small part of the complete testing cycle. Second and more importantly, running will not improve the productivity of the phlebotomists. They will not draw any more samples because they are already meeting existing demand levels. About all that will happen is that each phlebotomist will have three hours of idle time each day instead of two- and-one-half hours. The structural approach dictates the limits of productivity and even our ability to capture whatever "paper" gains we appear to achieve.

One more example is useful because it highlights not only the importance of the factors driving structural cost but also the role that service-level decisions play in limiting the potential for traditional productivity gains. Let us begin with a surprising statistic based on observations at multiple hospitals: the typical inpatient admitting clerk admits only about five or six patients per day. (If you find this hard to believe, check the numbers at your own hospital tomorrow morning.) How did this situation come to pass? Well, the way we staff the admitting office is based on service levels, not productivity. Furthermore, our structural decision to centralize the function and limit the job responsibilities of admitting clerks to just a few tasks (admitting and bed assignments) restricts the extent to which the clerks could be productive in the traditional sense of the word.

We did not staff the admitting office by estimating the average number of inpatient admissions per day, multiplying that number by the average number of minutes required to process an admission, and dividing by the number of minutes worked per clerical FTE. That would have been the classic approach, and it would have been totally inappropriate. More likely, the staffing in the admitting office was determined by some service imperative: for example, 95 percent of all patients to be admitted will wait twenty minutes or less to be processed. Then, using a queuing-theory model or a few days of observations, we determined the staffing needed to deliver that level of service. That is the right way to do it—assuming we are going to have a central admitting function. The fact that the average admitting clerk processes only five or six patients per day is therefore not the result of laziness or intentional lack of productivity. These jobs were explicitly designed with the knowledge that the clerks would be idle (but ready to work) 40 or 50 percent of the time.

We can see this same phenomenon in the way that banks use tellers. Three hours out of every four, a bank has more tellers than it needs. As customers, we almost never have this impression because most of our trips to the bank are on Fridays at lunch time (when everyone else also goes). We see the tellers busy and stretched to meet demand. The bank is usually forced to staff its windows to meet peak demand at a certain level of service—say, 95 percent of customers will wait in line five minutes or less. This inevitably leads to apparent overstaffing during most hours of the day. Productivity simply is not the issue.

As we proceed through the rest of this book, the primary emphasis will be on structural change. Although there is ore to be mined in examining the productivity level in hospitals and analyzing other cost inputs (for example, supplies and pharmaceuticals), these opportunities are dwarfed by those at the structural level. Furthermore, why should we concentrate our efforts on improving the execution of flawed processes that are full of potentially unnecessary work? As someone once said, "Anything not worth doing isn't worth doing right." Better to focus on changing the basic structure before we fine-tune the work steps we take for granted today.

Similar Hospital Operating Structures

Operating structures are especially critical in understanding the cost and service performance of hospitals. Virtually all hospitals have adopted the same operating approach. Viewed at the structural level, all hospitals are highly compartmentalized and fragmented, with specialized staff performing narrow tasks within the compartments. Figure 2.2 shows a highly schematic overview of a typical hospital operating structure.

Before describing the structure itself, we should remind ourselves of several facts. Remember that the average hospital has some one hundred or more activity centers. In fact, in large academic settings, the number can approach two hundred. These individual compartments are grouped into the four boxes shown

Figure 2.2. Schematic Operating Structure.

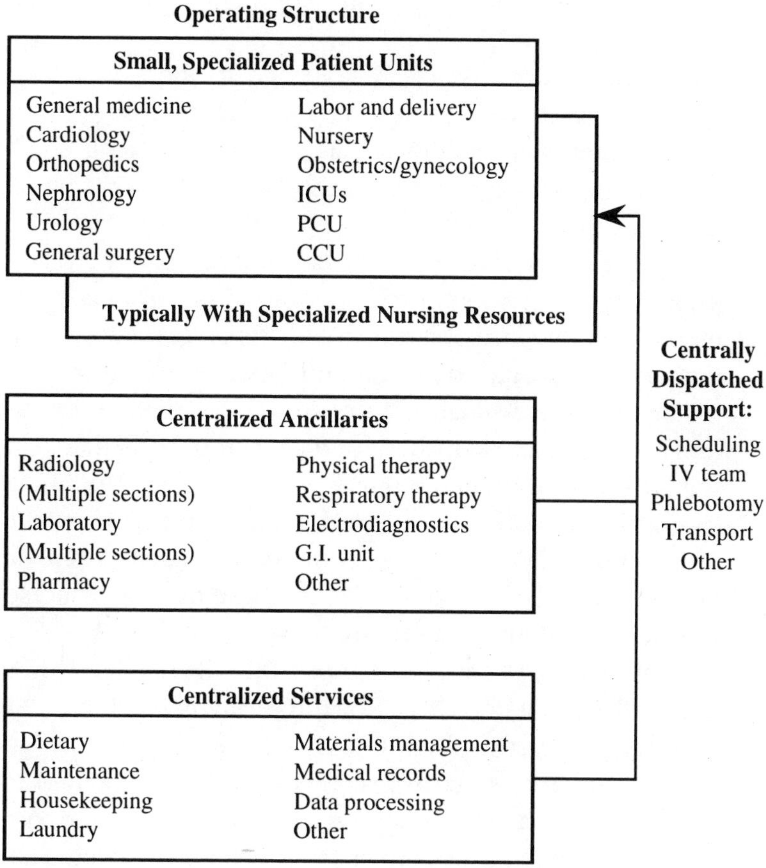

Operating Structure

Small, Specialized Patient Units	
General medicine	Labor and delivery
Cardiology	Nursery
Orthopedics	Obstetrics/gynecology
Nephrology	ICUs
Urology	PCU
General surgery	CCU

Typically With Specialized Nursing Resources

Centralized Ancillaries	
Radiology	Physical therapy
(Multiple sections)	Respiratory therapy
Laboratory	Electrodiagnostics
(Multiple sections)	G.I. unit
Pharmacy	Other

Centralized Services	
Dietary	Materials management
Maintenance	Medical records
Housekeeping	Data processing
Laundry	Other

Centrally Dispatched Support:
Scheduling
IV team
Phlebotomy
Transport
Other

on the left side of the graphic. The basic structure involves the following:

• There are numerous, relatively small patient care units (nursing units). The size of these is commonly between twenty-five and forty beds, with intensive care units (ICUs) often as small as six or eight beds. The units usually have a specific clinical focus: medicine, surgery, obstetrics, psychiatry, and so forth. In university hospitals, the distinctions can be even finer (medical oncology, surgical oncology) with no end in sight. Perhaps someday we will have a left retina unit and a right retina unit.

- Professional nursing staff are assigned to these units on a dedicated basis. With some exceptions at the margin, there is little interchangeability of nurses from unit to unit. Orthopedic nurses work only on orthopedics units, for example. Although the situation is changing with the advent of units integrating labor, delivery, recovery, and postpartum (LDRP), the ultimate extension of this specialization within compartments is the practice of having totally separate staffing for the nursery, the postpartum unit, and labor and delivery. This results in bizarre situations: the "mommie nurse" (postpartum) visits a patient in her room; if the baby is there and starts to cry, the mommie nurse is likely to run into the hall to find a "baby nurse" to care for the infant. This practice seems especially offensive to common sense, since one layperson (the mother) will tend to all these matters by herself within twenty-four hours or so.

- Hospitals have centralized virtually all ancillary functions—the laboratory, radiology, the pharmacy, EKG, EEG, respiratory therapy, physical and occupational therapy, and so forth. Selected services may be dispatched to the bedside (portable X rays and EKGs, for instance), but by and large we insist on moving the patient or a specimen to a central area for service. A natural outgrowth of this "action at a distance" is that elaborate scheduling and transportation work is needed to perform each function rendered centrally. As we will soon see, the hidden infrastructure costs of this approach are enormous.

- Service functions (including housekeeping, dietary, admitting, billing, medical records, maintenance, and the like) have also been thoroughly centralized. The most important result of this structural approach is the necessity of developing nearly uniform service levels throughout the hospital. For example, a centralized housekeeping service is usually constrained to a strict schedule: beds will be changed and rooms cleaned once a day, and the assembled masses of house-keepers will attempt to do that before noon (so they can clean common areas after lunch and be available for discharge and admission room changeovers).

To enable these one hundred or so organizational entities to communicate effectively and handle work involving multiple compartments of activity, we have had to invent all sorts of cen-trally dispatched and coordinated services—the glue holding the boxes together. These arrangements include scheduling systems, transporters, phlebotomists, and intravenous (IV) teams. Not even outpatient services are immune from this tendency. One large health maintenance organization (HMO) on the West Coast has an injection department in its larger primary care centers. Appar-ently their patients need yet another place to sit and wait for traditionally routine services.

No one is really to blame for the rapid proliferation of activity centers in the hospital. No one sat down and decided to create a mess. It resulted from hundreds and even thousands of incremental decisions—each seeming to make sense on its own terms but divorced from the larger picture of the overall opera-tion. In some cases, external forces had unintended side effects. For example, when Medicare in the early 1970s ruled that respira-tory care delivered by nurses could not be billed as a separate service, hospitals created or dramatically expanded their respira-tory therapy departments. The overwhelming proportion of their services was and continues to be relatively low-complexity proce-dures (intermitent positive-pressure breathing, spirometry, ox-imetry, oxygen therapy) that had previously been provided by the nursing staff. Now that Medicare (and other payers in increasing numbers) reimburse hospitals independent of charges, even that original expansion of routine services is called into question. The increased role of respiratory therapy in intensive care and other sophisticated services certainly argues the merits of its continued independent existence, but that does not mean that all services currently under its purview must be included in its mission throughout the hospital.

Excessive Staff Specialization

Compartmentalization goes much further than the proliferation of functions and activities. Staff specialization is the personal extension of the evolution of compartmentalization. Table 2.2 illustrates the proliferation of job classifications in the modern hospital; it shows a profile typical of a large community hospital. But even this data fails to dramatize the situation adequately. When we look a bit deeper, we find even more surprising evidence of the extent of specialization. Figure 2.3 presents a frequency distribution graph of job classifications in a large teaching hospital of about seven hundred beds. Nearly three-fourths of all job titles have fewer than five incumbents, and about one-half have just a single incumbent.

How did this situation come about? In part, the answer lies in hospitals' mimicking health care education. Increasing specialization throughout the past three decades has resulted in new disciplines in medicine as well as allied health professions (for example, sonographer, perfusionist). The possibility of generating a separate professional charge for billing purposes has also helped. The professions themselves also learned that most states were amenable to setting certification and registration standards. The proliferation and codification of these "guilds" continues to this day, encompassing not just nursing, medicine, and long-standing allied health professions but also phlebotomy and EKG in some states. Achieving guild status not only protects the public from unqualified practitioners—the usual justification— but is

Table 2.2. Job Classifications—Typical 500-Bed Hospital.

Category	Total
Job classes	350
Classes with fewer than ten employees	275
Average/class	6

Figure 2.3. Employees by Job Classification.

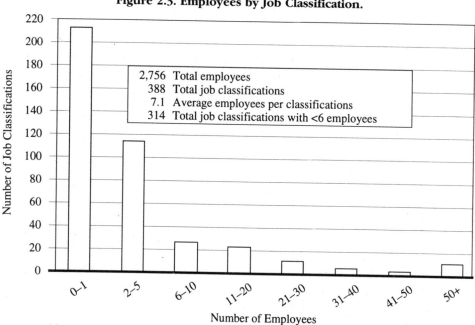

also a mechanism for enhancing job security by limiting the supply of potential staff members.

Even when such arguments make sense to the public, the regulators, and hospital executives, certification and training are often extended to define the work their practitioners will perform, rather than adding another qualification to an otherwise intelligent and motivated staff member. For example, nursing continues to pursue a path that seeks to define itself in ever-narrower terms: this activity is nursing; that activity is not. On one level, this is all well and good; we want highly qualified staff performing certain tasks. But the corollary of this trend is that nursing then makes the leap that it should perform *only* those tasks that are defined as nursing; anything else is demeaning to the profession. Furthermore, it is suggested, nurses are too expensive a resource to devote to anything other than their highest levels of activity. On paper, this thinking can sound reasonable, but its effect—applied throughout the hospital—is extreme compartmentalization, poor continuity of care, and high levels of idle time for staff members waiting for their jobs to be demanded.

To put this in perspective, let us try a management analogy. Let us say you are a senior executive with a graduate management degree (an M.B.A. or an M.H.A.). In the extreme professionalization framework, you might say to a subordinate, "Here, solve this simple equation for me. I'm an M.B.A., and I only perform calculus and multivariate analysis. You have a bachelor's degree in accounting, so you will perform my algebra for me." That employee in turn seeks out a clerk and says, "I only do algebra. When I need arithmetic done, I seek out a high school graduate like you to add up the numbers for me." This illustration should not be construed as arguing for nurses or other professionals to abandon their training and skills and become generic employees. But we do need to understand what has happened and that narrow job scopes (defined and limited to the highest level of skills attained) are part of the problem, not of the solution.

The nursing profession is certainly not alone in continuing to push the boundaries of education-defined jobs. A recent proposal by pharmacists is especially relevant. In the future, only doctorate-level programs will be accredited as preparation for hospital practice. Is this requirement really addressing the problems of hospital pharmacy services? Is the problem today that the disembodied voice at the other end of the phone with a physician does not have doctoral qualifications? We may never know if we keep today's operating structure. Although many hospital pharmacies continue to decentralize via satellites and assigned floor pharmacists, they continue the fragmentation of services. For example, satellite pharmacies often fill only initial orders. Daily refills and IV therapy are handled by others. Thus, the idea of getting pharmacists out on the floors and closer to doctors and care givers may be laudable, but the role can remain fragmented and discontinuous. Perhaps we should first pursue the decentralized model more aggressively—redeploying full pharmacy services—before redefining the qualifications of professionals too often buried in their hospital's compartmentalized structure.

Hospitals have aided and abetted these developments. Not only do most professionals gain status with their peers through increased specialization, hospitals reward them with more pay. In a sense, this system is entirely appropriate. We should reward new skills when they bring additional value to the organization and its patients. The problem is that greater specialization has become virtually the *only* way to increase the real compensation of many professional and technical staff members. There is one other way, of course; jump into management—on the theory that if you are good at performing a given function, you will be good at managing that function. The development of "clinical ladders" in recent years contains an element of the answer in their rationale but remains focused on increasing functional depth, with few features likely to inspire the development of broader skills. In the future, we will need compensation systems that for most employees encourage greater breadth, while continuing to provide incentives for some to enrich their functional depth.

This section would not be complete without at least one example of the inadvertent flexibility and compromise that the current system demonstrates every so often. The clinical laboratory at most hospitals is heavily staffed during the day shift and for good reason; that is when two-thirds or more of the demand occurs. During the day shift, each section of the lab (hematology, chemistry, microbiology) is staffed by full-time specialists, sometimes even dedicated to particular machines. It would be unusual in any but the most progressive of labs for microbiology staff members on this shift to walk across the hall during a slow period and offer to help the staff of a busier section. This is partly because throughput is often limited by the number of machines available, not number of staff members. The other reason is the outgrowth of compartmentalization and specialization. The lab staff members are made to feel accountable for a specific bundle of tasks assigned to their particular compartment, not laboratory service overall. Furthermore, their productivity measurements will not look any better if they help out another section. These attitudes are not mean spirited, merely a result of the structure. Curiously, however, by the time the evening and night shifts roll around, the entire laboratory is staffed by a small crew of generalists. The fact that most people do not like to work these shifts seems to break down many of the specialization barriers. A similar breakdown in the rigid roles of the day shift occurs routinely for nurses working offshifts; they frequently draw blood samples, start IVs, and perform EKGs and a variety of other tasks deemed professionally sacrosanct during the more popular shifts.

The compartmentalization of the modern hospital is continuing. In conjunction with its corollary (staff specialization), hospitals are coming to resemble the industrial models of past decades. Although this result is in large part unintentional, it is almost certainly inappropriate for the majority of hospital services. Manufacturing models based on assembly lines staffed with workers performing the same tasks hundreds of times a day are not an appropriate analog for a service business, much less one that is complex and highly customized. The idea in manufacturing was to "idiotproof" jobs so that little training was required, and the workers could be interchangeable on short notice. Through standardization, exceptions to the norm would be rare indeed. None of these principles applies to a service business or a hospital, especially the notion that exceptions to the norm are rare. The essence of a service business is its variability, particularly in health care. Rigid and multilayered hierarchies are the arch enemies of customer service and responsiveness. Exceptions *are* the norm, and front-line employees must be capable of dealing with a wide range of variability without mandatory recourse to a complex, vertical network of parallel, layered management structures. Once a customer's problem enters that bureaucracy, the service opportunity is irretrievably lost.

3

Compartmentalization

and Its Discontents:

High Cost and

Poor Service

Now is the time to introduce process flow charts and marvel at the complexity that our current organization structures inflict on our patients, doctors, and staffs. We will do this in due course. But if we step back and remind ourselves that we are dealing with services to human beings (often who are in discomfort or distress), a better starting point for understanding the problems of compartmentalization is to tell the story of an average patient undergoing a routine procedure. All the shortcomings of the system appear in sharp relief, features commonly lost in the clutter of flow charts.

A "Simple" Chest Film?

Let us see how the modern hospital goes about delivering one of its highest volume procedures: a chest X ray. Chest X rays account for upwards of 50 percent of all inpatient demand for general diagnostic radiology. You would think we would have it down to a fine science. We do not. Here, without much exaggeration, is the initial sequence of major events required in most hospitals today:

- The doctor is on rounds and asks the nurse to arrange for the patient, Mr. Smith, to get a chest film today.
- The nurse duly records the order in Mr. Smith's chart. Some time later, the nurse transmits this request to the ward secretary, who writes it down.
- Some time later, the ward secretary calls radiology to schedule the procedure for Room 4 at 3:05 P.M. Someone in radiology and the ward secretary both write it down.
- The ward secretary then calls transportation to arrange to get Mr. Smith to radiology by 3:05 P.M. The transportation scheduler tells the ward secretary that Bob will get Mr. Smith at 2:50. The transportation scheduler and the ward secretary both write down this information.
- Bob, if he is an experienced transporter, will call the unit before he begins his journey. There is a 25 percent probability Mr. Smith will be nowhere near his room at 2:50 P.M.
- After confirming Mr. Smith's availability, Bob begins his trek. He finds an elevator bank, pushes the button, and waits for an elevator.
- When the elevator deposits him on the right floor, he goes to the nursing station to find Mr. Smith's chart—if it is there. He then must have a documented hand-off from nursing. Nursing will note that Mr. Smith was alive when they released him to Bob, and Bob may also make an entry. Mr. Smith will be handed off so many times that we need to know who to blame if something goes wrong and also because we want to record how busy everyone is.
- Bob then goes to Mr. Smith's room and puts him in a wheelchair (if he can find one) for the trip.
- They go to the elevator bank and wait, ride down to radiology, get off the elevator, and proceed down the hall, right to the threshold of the X ray department.

- Bob notifies the radiology receptionist that Mr. Smith has arrived for his chest film and hands over the chart. The receptionist logs Mr. Smith in. And then . . .

Freeze the frame on this little movie. To review the process so far, the hospital has just succeeded in having six members of its staff flawlessly execute thirty or forty minutes of work that management designed for them to do—in fact, pays them well to do many times a day. And what has actually happened? Nothing. Nothing has taken place that is clinically important or contributes to the quality of the chest film that was ordered for Mr. Smith. All of this was simply work necessitated by our decision to perform routine X rays in one central location and to utilize the services of a central pool of transportation aides. Was our staff "productive" in the performance of these duties? Yes. Will each activity be duly recorded somewhere in our productivity monitoring system? Of course. Did the patient or the physician get good service? Hardly.

Oh, by the way, we will have to repeat this process to get Mr. Smith back to his room. And why do we do this? Why do we roll Mr. Smith all over the hospital for two hours (clad in his institutional pajamas) and make him unavailable for any other procedures or activities (like lunch) while all this is going on? To do a chest film. A chest film involves about three to five minutes of a technologist's time and the average radiologist reads the average chest film in less than thirty seconds! And let us not forget the attending physician in all this. The requesting physician is likely to wait at least four hours to get the results of this consultation.

The situation can actually be even more extreme, as in the case of transporting patients to a central area for EKGs. Relatively few hospitals still do this, thankfully, but it is perhaps the ultimate example of compartmentalization and specialization run amok. Most of the scheduling and transportation work just described for an X ray must also be done to arrange a centralized EKG. But here the triumph of process over content is even more complete. After all, what is involved in an EKG? A machine costing $2,000

or $3,000 that has the color-coded instructions on the lid, oper-
ated by an employee who came to the hospital with nothing more
than a high school diploma and a willingness to learn. Such an
employee can be trained to do EKGs in a matter of a few weeks.
Of course, we do not mean to denigrate the work of EKG technicians. They do what they have been asked to do and do it well.
It is the structure that creates the low value that is actually produced by all the work needed to accomplish such straightforward
tasks.

　　These are the true penalties of compartmentalization: the
high cost of arranging and keeping track of all the discrete tasks
we do and the resulting poor service levels we are doomed to
provide. The following sections present a more scientific analysis
of these factors and pursue their implications.

Process Complexity

Now let us reexamine the inpatient X ray process in more detail
and include the activities that occur behind the scenes—file
preparation, transcription, and so forth. Figure 3.1 identifies all
the steps involved in providing an inpatient chest film. In Booz •
Allen's work with more than two dozen hospitals, the X ray process always looks about the same. Forty or more work steps seem
to be the normal course of events. For those of you who lack the
patience or interest to examine the flow chart in detail, rest assured that the enumerated steps are real and not contrived to
make the point. Phoning to schedule the procedure, for instance,
is one work step; we have not counted each digit of the dialing
process.

　　The flow chart is perhaps best used by ophthalmologists
to check for farsightedness. A more useful summary is presented
in Table 3.1.

　　The entire process involves forty steps (although the number can be as high as sixty) and requires over two hours of process
time. Let us be clear about this: process time is *work*, not total
turnaround time, which is generally four hours or more. Many

Table 3.1. Radiology Process Summary.

	Steps	Minutes
Medical-clinical activities	6	21
Transportation	8	42
Communication and coordination	12	26
Clerical tasks including data entry	14	51
Total	40	140

attending physicians will therefore go to radiology themselves to review crucial films on the viewing box before the formal consult is completed. Depending on the institution, twelve to fifteen different staff members can be involved in the process from start to finish.

The precise number of work steps is neither here nor there; the important point is to look at what is being done. A chest film entails a few minutes of a technologist's time and less than a minute of a radiologist's reading time. The chart shows a total of six steps and twenty minutes for medical-technical-clinical work. This allotment is a bit generous and includes the possibility that the patient requires some physical assistance, the technologist reviews the chart at a high level, and/or the radiologist compares the film to earlier films for the same patient. Even so, only about 15 percent of the overall process is devoted to activities directly involved in the clinical content of the procedure.

What else is going on here? Look at the number of work steps and amount of time devoted to scheduling and coordination activities, work that is created by our structural decisions to centralize routine radiology. Nearly 30 percent of the process is consumed by this work. In many cases, its real benefits are hard to find. Think about your own hospital. It is very likely that if you set out to visit the radiology department at, say, 8:00 A.M., you would know you were getting close to the department before you actually arrived at the door. Why? Because you would see a line of patients on gurneys or in wheelchairs. Each of these patients is likely to have a precisely scheduled appointment for a

Figure 3.1. Routine Radiology Work Flow: Typical Diagnostic X ray Process.

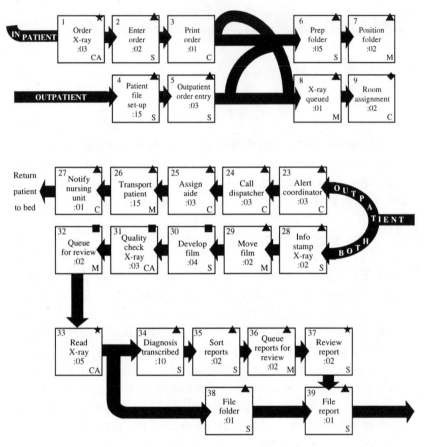

Figure 3.1. Routine Radiology Work Flow: Typical Diagnostic X ray Process. Cont'd.

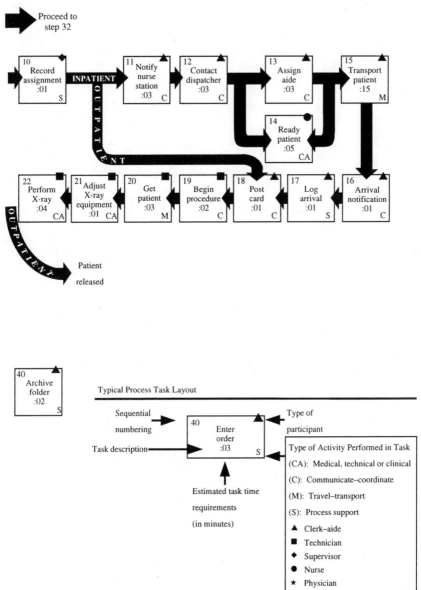

Figure 3.2. Laboratory Test Process Flow.

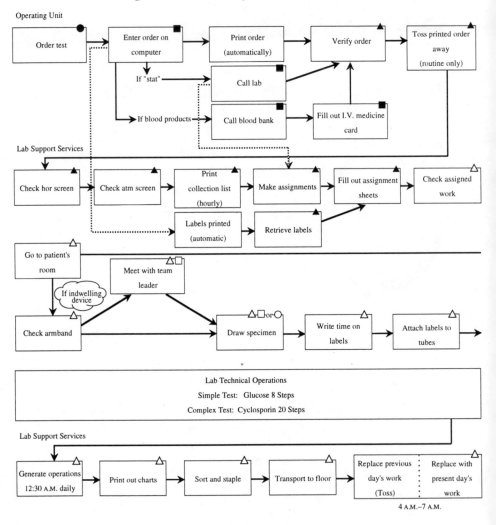

Figure 3.2. Laboratory Test Process Flow. Cont'd.

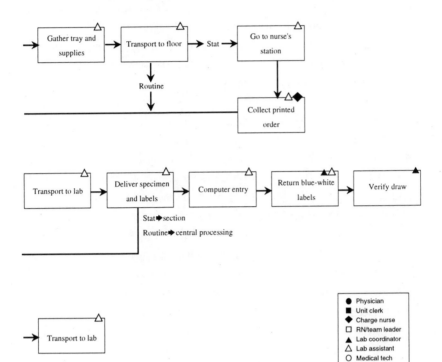

general radiology procedure; yet there they wait. Our big investment in scheduling this work does not seem to pay off for patients or their physicians during peak periods.

One hospital decided to see if there were major benefits to all this precise scheduling of routine procedures. A quick bit of queuing analysis gave a surprising result: the line of gurneys and wheelchairs at peak demand periods would not be any worse if we did not schedule routine radiology procedures at all. Even a low-tech scheduling system would be oversophisticated. For instance, we could install a switch at the radiology reception desk. When the receptionist counted three or more patients in line, she would throw the switch. This action would activate a red light at each nursing station, signaling that no more routine radiology patients should be sent down until the light went off. But this innovation would be technological overkill since the light would almost certainly go off in three or four minutes. It is likely that all our scheduling is driven by a desire to engage our technologists and machines fully in advance and to even up the day's work more than by a desire to minimize inconvenience to patients.

This level of complexity is not confined to procedures requiring the presence of the patient. The laboratory exhibits similar behavior, with an especially interesting twist. Figure 3.2 presents the work steps and flow involved in getting a straightforward laboratory test on a routine order basis (not stat). Buried in the middle of this mess is an elongated box labeled "perform test." Virtually all of the work depicted in the other thirty or so boxes is generic in nature and does not vary significantly, regardless of the test that is requested. Here is a case where the infrastructure clearly dominates the work. This example points to the futility of many efforts to improve or streamline the process. It also should make us question our usual preoccupation with reagent cost and machine throughput when making decisions about laboratory work. These are simply not the key issues in overall cost or responsiveness.

The Futility of Incremental Change

It is hard to see how we can take the X ray process and make substantial improvements within the existing model. What usually happens is that a hospital will sense a problem with, say, radiology service levels and put a team to work on it. This team will work diligently for several months and issue a report that in essence declares victory: "We have reduced the number of steps required from forty to thirty-three and eliminated fourteen minutes of process time." The problem is that this sort of incremental change will not be noticed by patients or their physicians, and the CFO will not be able to find the savings with a microscope. The eliminated steps and process time will simply fall into the hospitalwide black hole of idle time. We might succeed in saving fifteen or twenty minutes per day for twenty different employees but cannot translate this into the elimination of a single FTE. Our processes today are simply too complex and related to other activities to allow us to benefit from isolated, incremental improvements in any given function.

This fact is a particular challenge for institutions that have embarked on major TQM or CQI programs. Each set of concepts is valid and useful, but in and of themselves they are merely processes in search of an idea. Each needs a vision that guides and prioritizes its execution. To send out armies of TQM teams to find and solve their own problems is an exercise in futility. Such teams will seldom, if ever, come back to top management and say, "The problem is that our jobs would not be necessary if we could reengineer such-and-such process. Furthermore, Departments *C* and *D* could be eliminated or absorbed into Department *E*." These kinds of fundamental change are simply not conceivable. By contrast, if a TQM process were launched with one overarching goal—improving continuity of care by reducing the number of employees who interact with each patient, say—the teams would be forced to confront the underlying issues. Incremental change would obviously not be the dominant means of improvement.

"Competition" for Patients

Hospitals are accustomed to thinking about competition in terms of interinstitutional struggles for market share and physicians. Unfortunately, our internal operating structures produce an unintended form of competition for patients. Each patient's day is a complicated and orchestrated series of transactions. Most of these involve a staff member being dispatched from a central location or the patient being transported to a centralized service. The computer system has not been designed that can track all of these movements for a patient, much less handle the variability of each individual procedure. Consequently, we simply try to do our best to get everything done—scheduling those things that can (or must) be scheduled and hoping for the best in all the other transactions (meals, phlebotomy, medications, vital signs, and the like).

Recall Mr. Smith's X ray experience. One of the uncertainties was whether Mr. Smith would actually be in his room when the transporter arrived at the appointed time to move him to radiology. A good rule of thumb is that this expectation is met only about 75 percent of the time. And this is for a scheduled procedure. When the procedure is unscheduled (or only specified to occur within, say, a four-hour window of time), the predictability decreases even more dramatically.

Figure 3.3 presents the picture of respiratory therapists making their rounds for routine procedures. This chart shows that a therapist succeeds only about half of the time on the first attempt to provide care. There are a variety of competing transactions and contributing conditions. The patient is not in the room—perhaps delayed in his return from radiology or physical therapy. The patient is in the bathroom or taking a shower. The attending physician is present and does not wish to be disturbed. Nursing is performing a treatment that should not be interrupted (for example, a dressing change). It requires an average of three visits to deliver two respiratory therapy treatments. Where is this built-in, 33 percent inefficiency accounted for in our productivity

Figure 3.3. "Competition" for Patients.

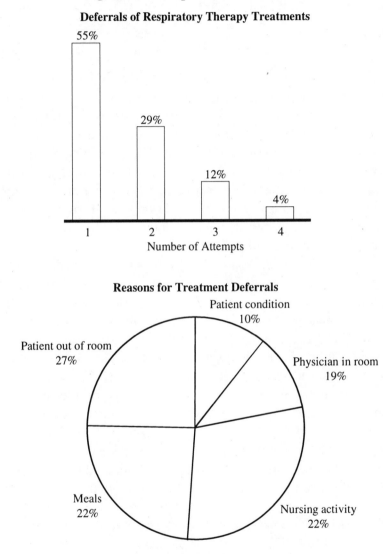

Deferrals of Respiratory Therapy Treatments

Reasons for Treatment Deferrals

Number of Treatments = 91

systems? Nowhere. Yet our operating structure makes this problem nearly unavoidable and holds the therapists accountable for how they spend their time and our money.

Structural Idle Time

It is time to give a name to a concept that has infiltrated virtually every dimension of the discussion so far: *structural idle time.* Structural idle time refers to lost productive time but is not productivity per se. For example, if you are told that your job is to shovel dirt and your supervisor comes by to check on you and finds you leaning on your shovel, the supervisor has a very straightforward productivity problem with you. But if you are told that your job is to answer the phone when it rings, you are structurally idle if your supervisor finds you doing nothing but the phone is not ringing. The difference is that your job was not designed to give you something to do when the phone is not ringing—documents to file, envelopes to stuff, numbers to add up or whatever. Almost every job in the world has structural idle time. Hospital jobs tend to have extraordinary amounts of it.

The sources of structural idle time in hospitals are compartmentalization, specialization, and demand variability. We have already covered the compartmentalization and specialization dimensions in some detail. Recall that the average hospital has over one hundred activity centers, each with fairly narrow service missions. Within these centers are specialized staff members with very narrow job descriptions. When these factors are compounded by the highly variable nature of demand for individual hospital procedures, the result is structural idle time with a vengeance.

Hospital demand follows four general patterns: haphazard, forecastable, predictable, and "schedulable"—each reflecting an increased level of precision. The lines of differentiation between these categories are not always crystal clear, but we need to understand what each one means and its effect on operating performance.

- Haphazard demand is nearly self-explanatory and includes mostly near-term, seemingly random variations in activity levels. In fact, if we choose a sufficiently distant planning horizon, very little demand is truly haphazard. Although we cannot forecast a specific multicar accident arriving in our emergency department, we can be reasonably certain that during a given one-year period we will have, say, five such incidents to deal with. What separates haphazard demand from the other categories is that it is useless to invest time trying to predict or forecast this demand.

- Forecastable demand provides a useful level of certainty over a given planning horizon. This is the level most hospital managers are most accustomed to dealing with. Most budgeting numbers are forecasts; they seek to estimate fairly gross demand levels, such as annual admissions or patient days, quarterly RVU demand in the hematology section of the lab, and total number of outpatient surgeries. At this level, forecasting is a useful tool for estimating total resource requirements over a reasonably long period of time.

- Predictable demand deals with shorter planning horizons and greater specificity than forecasts. For instance, for a specific admission (a colectomy, say), we can accurately predict what will be done for the majority of uncomplicated cases. They will stay four days, spend two hours or so in the operating room, get one postsurgical chest X ray, start on a regular diet three days postoperatively, and so forth. At a slightly higher level, we can predict with accuracy the total number of CBCs we will do when the census is at 233 patients. The predictability of demand is often intuited by experienced employees, rather than codified into any specific system. Even before critical pathways were invented, most surgeons had standing preop and postop orders, and most experienced nurses could predict patient needs from hour to hour and day to day. This is probably the least exploited level of formal demand anticipation in hospitals today.

- "Schedulability" is also a fairly self-explanatory concept. This is where we translate a particular forecastable or predictable activity into a precisely scheduled event. Running down the hierarchy in a specific example, we expect 240 colectomies this year (forecast); each colectomy will require two hours in the operating room (prediction); and Mrs. Johnson will have her colectomy next Thursday from 7:00 A.M. to 9:00 A.M. (schedule).

The current operating structure makes it very difficult to respond effectively to variations in demand, even when we can predict or forecast them. In general, we set up a forecasted level of demand, provide the resources to meet that demand in gross terms, and then hope for the best. We are essentially in a fixed-cost environment within broad limits of demand variability. For example, assume a hospital has a census today of 250 patients. Wave a magic wand, and make that number 230 patients. What changes in terms of cost? Virtually nothing. We do not send home 8 percent of the staff or spend 8 percent less on food. The system just is not that precise or responsive. Similarly, if you wave your magic wand and make the census 270 today, we do not add to the staff or send out a rush order for more food. About the only thing that changes under either of these scenarios is the revenue line. For hospitals, there is probably truth in the cynical aphorism, "costs are fixed as volume goes down and variable as volume increases."

The real problem is that there is no lack of variation in demand in hospitals—from season to season, from week to week, from shift to shift, even from hour to hour. For the most part, we are helpless to respond with well-timed changes in the resources devoted to the tasks (beyond perhaps authorizing overtime or bringing in more agency personnel—both actions targeted at meeting increases in demand, not responding to declines). Elegant nurse-staffing systems consume lots of time and expense gathering data for each shift, but they do little more than an experienced eye and common sense could achieve in ten minutes of analysis. This is the problem with many such tools; they try to manage outcomes without any control over demand. The difference between good performance and bad is often an accident of that day's demand level. Further, our rigid organization structures make idle time in one area (driven by demand variability) unavailable to fill gaps in other areas. Consequently, we tend to staff all organizational compartments for their near-peak demand levels. This approach compounds the already considerable problem of structural idle time in hospitals.

As we will see in later chapters, the solution to this problem is not in general to seek ever more sophisticated forecasting capabilities but rather to restructure work so that our staff members can be more independently and broadly responsive to changes in demand. We will restructure to create fewer but larger and more flexible compartments of fixed cost.

Hospitalwide Value Added—How We Spend Our Time

It should be very clear at this point that the road to insight and improvement is not going to lead us directly inside the hundred or so organizational boxes. Trying to optimize the performance of each cost center on the Medicare cost report is what got us into this situation in the first place. It is time to ask a seemingly naive and deceptively simple question: what do people do in our hospitals? In other words, how do they spend their time and our resources in the course of working within the operating structures we designed? We also want to avoid the temptation to get overly microscopic at this stage, to lose sight of the overall picture by getting mired in fine distinctions. That level of detail can come later, after we have seen the larger workings of the structure in sharp relief.

To this end, we developed nine categories of activity to evaluate and estimate. They are almost obvious and merely describe the general nature of the work being performed. We could define additional categories, but it seems unlikely that any greater insight or benefit would accrue. The nine categories are described as follows:

- *Medical-technical-clinical tasks*—what we all think of as "health care." This category includes both procedure-specific work and cognitive activities. Procedures include everything from drawing blood and taking vital signs, to performing a CAT scan and inserting a central line. Cognitive work includes care planning, counseling, patient education, and assessments. These are the services people come to a hospital or a clinic to obtain and to which they expect the bulk of institutional resources to be devoted.

- *Hotel services*—essentially the work needed to feed patients and keep their rooms and beds clean and fresh. It also includes the upkeep and maintenance of the facilities and equipment.

- *Medical documentation* —everything that goes into writing down clinical information or information associated with clinical activities. Notations in the chart, results from the lab, nursing care plans, and discharge summaries fall into this category.

- *Institutional documentation* —all the documentation work not directly associated with clinical activities. Examples include memos, time cards, budgets, financial reports, and employee evaluations.

- *Scheduling and coordinating* —the time spent arranging to do the work of the hospital. Recall all the scheduling transactions involved in an X ray, the endless calls to various departments, the level loading of respiratory work on a shift, and so forth. Also included here are the hundreds of calls nurses make every day simply trying to find their patients in the system or to expedite their progress from point to point.

- *Patient transportation* —moving patients to and from their rooms for various services in the hospital, including escort of patients to their rooms upon admission and to the front door for discharge.

- *Staff transportation* —staff members going from work site to work site and also their movement to assemble the proper supplies and equipment at the right location.

- *Management and supervision* —the time involved in typical management tasks. This affects both staff members designated as full-time managers and supervisors and a portion of non-management staffers in their roles as "player-coaches."
- *Ready for action*—a somewhat kinder and gentler rubric for "structural idle time." This category consists of the time our staffs spend waiting for their specific jobs to be demanded or waiting for others to complete their three or four steps of a forty-step process. Ready-for-action time is not automatically inappropriate. In fact, in service businesses, it is a necessary part of the enterprise. This is doubly true in any service with an emergency component. Just as we would not want our fire department to have zero ready-for-action time (especially if *our* house should be the next to catch fire), so hospitals must build in a certain amount of ready-for-action time. The important question is, of course, how much?

Figure 3.4 presents the results of the value-added analysis for a typical hospital of two hundred beds or more. The numbers show the percent of personnel time and cost devoted to each category of the value-added structure. In more than two dozen iterations of this work for hospitals of 200 to 750 beds, the results are remarkably similar. Individual components vary by no more than a few percentage points from institution to institution. This outcome probably should not be surprising, given that almost all hospitals have the same operating structure.

Before discussing the magnitudes of the individual components, a few qualifying remarks are necessary. First, the methodology involved estimates based on selected observations of employees and interviews with staff and supervisors. Not every employee was observed, but key positions were monitored and their activities recorded. Second, this was not a mere allocation of time by type of position—that is, not all of a nurse's time was allocated as medical-technical-clinical work. There were actual observations of how much time was spent running for supplies, documenting care, counseling patients and staff members, and so

Figure 3.4. Value-Added Profile: Percentage of Personnel Time and Cost Devoted to Activities.

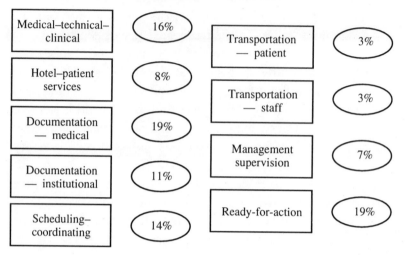

forth; moreover, these components could vary significantly by the level (head nurse, team leader, and so forth) and type of nurse (critical care, maternity, surgical). Further, the analysis was probably generous in some regards. For instance, consider a cardiac monitoring technician. Though most of this job can consist of watching monitors and looking for problems and alarms, not all such work was classified as ready-for-action time. The content of the job was deemed to be clinical and technical because its very essence was to be ready for a very specific clinical situation.

Overall, the results were stunning and troubling. Fewer than twenty cents on the dollar was devoted to the direct care of patients. Even adding in the hotel component (8 percent) only raised the total to 24 percent. A nearly equal amount of time (14 percent) was devoted to scheduling and arranging the care actually provided. Nineteen percent of the value added consisted of structural idle time. In a vivid demonstration of the dominance of clerical work, 30 percent of personnel time is spent writing things down, and most of that is clinically related documentation.

To state the situation a bit more bluntly: for every dollar spent on something that is visible to customers, three or four dollars is spent on infrastructure costs.

It is as if a group of futurists sat in a conference center twenty years ago trying to envision the hospital of the future. After weeks of deliberation, this august body gave up on the whole idea, except to announce to the waiting world two general rules all hospitals should eventually follow. First, the hospital should devote no more than 20 percent of its efforts to direct patient care activities. Second, every patient has the inalienable right to meet fifteen different employees during each day of stay. It did not happen this way, of course, and there is no gaggle of gurus to blame our troubles on. Nevertheless, those facts do not change the mess we are in.

Just as we saw with the complicated X ray process, it is almost impossible to imagine how a series of incremental changes will fundamentally alter the current value-added structure. Ten percent improvements in selected value-added components would have only minimal effects on the absolute amount of time and money devoted to various infrastructure items. We need to open ourselves to dramatic changes that not only refocus institutional resources but also succeed in improving services to customers and the costs we all incur. This is the only way in which value is truly delivered.

Even at this early stage in the analysis, a few directional guidelines about the transition to a new world are possible. Our first concern should be changing *where* and *how* resources are spent, rather than worrying about the total amount of resources involved. Yes, cost reduction is a goal, but if we cannot improve the percentage of resources devoted to direct care, we will not have had a profound effect on what truly ails our system today. To illustrate this point, one hospital speculated very early that it could improve patient service and satisfaction without restructuring. All the seating surfaces on a nursing unit could be ripped out and replaced with chairs bolted to the floors of patient rooms.

Even if this did not reduce nursing documentation time and idle time, at least it would encourage most of this time to be spent in contact with patients (instead of other employees). This was never a serious suggestion; it was intended as a useful exercise in understanding what the challenge was really all about.

We can also speculate about the dislocations that we are likely to cause by seeking to increase the percentages of our value added that are devoted to direct care and service. People who are now primarily involved in writing things down, moving things through the hospital, scheduling activities, and managing narrow functional groupings are going to find their lives changing dramatically. To the extent we reduce total cost, many of these people will be displaced over time. More importantly, though, they will find the content of their work changing, both in scope and focus. Retraining and attrition will ultimately make room for most of these staff members. The group at greatest risk in the long run will be middle managers, many of whose jobs will go away with the flattening of the organization and whose opportunities for fitting into the new structure at their current pay levels will be limited.

None of these implications should deter us from pushing the concepts forward. But just as we need to look to the human needs of our patients, we need to be aware of the personal impact we will have on our work force. Restructuring is not just a scary prospect for a corporation, it will be an anxious journey for everyone in the organization. This dimension is likely to cause stress within the organization more than any of the technical challenges involved.

4

Patient Focus

Begins with Demand

Almost all of our journey so far has focused on the supply side of the hospital operations equation. We have examined what the hospital does (chest films, for instance) in terms of the processes used, the people involved, and the resources devoted to the effort. How these services came to be demanded in the first place has not been our concern. Nor have the patterns and clusters of demand been analyzed for their operating implications. These issues are the subject of this chapter. If we are going to move forward in the name of service to our patients, the demand side of the equation must be our starting off point. In restructuring service businesses, it is our customers' needs that should shape the basic operating approach.

One Size Fits None

The similarity of hospital operating structures that we saw earlier has a corollary within hospital functions themselves. Just as there appears to be a one-size-fits-all paradigm for the design of hospital operations across geographies, missions, and sizes, there is a similar approach to the services provided by individual departments and sections. Worse yet, the approach is seemingly built around a highest-common-denominator mentality. In essence, hospitals seem to have designed their operations around the following baseline parameters: describe the busiest time on the busiest day of the year; then add to that demand the sickest possible patient with the most complex set of needs; then design operations to meet that standard at all times. Unfortunately, these notions are misguided and leave significant service and cost opportunities on the table. We serve neither our customers' best interests nor our own by adopting this kind of operating strategy.

To illustrate this point, let us again imagine that we are sitting in a conference center twenty years ago trying to plan the hospital of the future. We begin this process—logically enough—by characterizing the nature of patient care needs with which our customers will present us. Only then can we begin to structure our operating approach. In this imaginary exercise, we allow ourselves the expedient of oversimplifying the problem. We will deal with only two types of somewhat idealized patients: general surgery patients and medical diagnostic ones. Figure 4.1 summarizes the key characteristics of each patient category.

Figure 4.1. Operational Challenges.

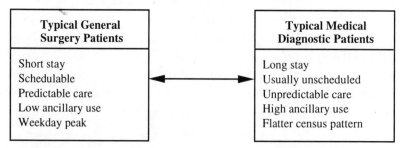

Typical General Surgery Patients	Typical Medical Diagnostic Patients
Short stay Schedulable Predictable care Low ancillary use Weekday peak	Long stay Usually unscheduled Unpredictable care High ancillary use Flatter census pattern

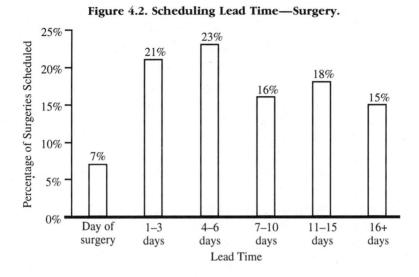

Figure 4.2. Scheduling Lead Time—Surgery.

Let us examine in some detail the operational challenges with which each kind of patient will confront us. First, there are our surgical customers.

- Short stays predominate—two, three, or four days in most cases.
- These patients are generally "schedulable." It is common to find 70 percent or more of these cases scheduled at least three days in advance, as shown in Figure 4.2.
- The postsurgical care of these patients is highly predictable. We know almost hour by hour what these patients are likely to need from the time they return from surgery until they are discharged. This situation is nearly as true for open-heart surgery as it is for gallbladder surgery.
- These patients consume relatively few ancillary services postoperatively. When they do need them, it is generally from the lower-complexity end of the spectrum—electrolytes, chest films, and spirometry, for example.

- Because of these patients' short stays and surgeons' scheduling preferences, we usually see a weekday peak in the census and a bit of a lull on weekends.

    Well, what about medical diagnostic patients? Do they exhibit these same kinds of features and patterns in their needs? Of course not.

- Medicine patients' stays are much longer—eight, ten, sixteen days.
- They are generally unscheduled. The first we know of them is when they present in a physician's office or the emergency room with something numb or something bleeding where we cannot see it. Many are admitted on an urgent or emergency basis.
- Their care is often unpredictable, and the course of their treatment and recovery fraught with branchings, plateaus, and monitored responses to various options.
- At the same time, they are likely to consume reasonably high levels of our most sophisticated ancillary services during their first forty-eight hours of hospitalization. In addition to outpatients, the primary consumers of MRIs, CAT scans, and nuclear medicine procedures are medicine patients during the diagnostic (front-end) portions of their stays.
- Because of the less predictable nature of demand and the longer stays involved, this group's census tends to show less dramatic swings from weekdays to weekends.

    Exaggerating only slightly to make the point, the only distinction hospitals now make between these fundamentally different sets of customer needs is the kind of nurse patients get and the number of hours a day. For example, surgical patients get 4.3 hours per day of nursing care. Medical patients receive 3.9 hours. If this seems an unfair or even a cruel caricature, it is more true than you would think. The way that these patients get admitted, have their drugs ordered, have their charts documented, receive their meals, get their X rays and lab work, and have their rooms cleaned is the same for all of them. One size fits all. Take it or leave it.

Let us look at a few examples to see what the one-size-fits-all approach actually delivers in terms of customer service. As a rule, it will usually result in overserving some customers' needs and underserving those of others. Consider housekeeping. The standard operating structure and approach for this function in hospitals today is a single, centralized service. What this means is that at about 6:00 or 7:00 A.M. every day, forty or fifty house-keepers arrive on the scene and must be kept "productive." These employees therefore fan out to their appointed duty areas and attempt to clean all occupied patient rooms before lunch. After lunch, their duties change somewhat; a portion are assigned to cleaning common areas, and a portion are kept on call to process room turnovers (discharges and admissions). This approach best keeps the centralized pool of housekeepers working. Scheduling and "routes" are critical to this operating structure because there is virtually nothing else these employees are trained and positioned to do.

But what does this operating structure say to patients—our customers? It says that they may only get their beds changed once a day under normal circumstances. No one asked the patient if once a day was the right frequency for linen changes. It is probably entirely appropriate in a hotel; however, hospital patients do not merely sleep in their beds, they live in them. Even if once a day were the absolute best we could do for our patients, no one asked them if the morning would be the best or most convenient time to change their beds. It is entirely likely that many, reckoning evening to be the time of day that a clean set of bed linens would provide the greatest pleasure and benefit, would opt to have their beds changed then. Yet our one-size-fits-all approach cannot begin to respond to any demand as amorphous and unpredictable as this. We change beds once a day—in the morning—because our large, single-task work force of housekeepers finds this the easiest standard to meet while striving to remain productive.

Let us now consider a different example, using somewhat different groups of patients. Consider the coding of medical records for billing purposes. How is this procedure done today? For the most part, all charts are sent to somewhere in medical records shortly after the patient is discharged. Here they languish for several days, waiting for various loose sheets to trickle down (generally lab reports and X ray consultations from the last day or two of the patient's stay). The records and loose sheets are put together with the discharge summary by someone completely unfamiliar with the patient and the care givers who then attempts to assign the correct code. The primary usefulness of this process to the hospital is to get the proper payment; higher-minded purposes of quality assurance and record completeness are secondary. The result of this standardized approach is uneven and disproportionate service to various patient groups, as well as high cost. Let us examine the coding needs of two types of patients.

Obstetrics patients. It only takes about eight diagnosis-related groupings (DRGs) to account for more than 90 percent of their conditions. Furthermore, the distinctions between the diagnoses are not subtle, and the nurses involved in their care will get the right answer 95 percent of the time (they are unlikely ever to get the wrong answer; the remaining 5 percent are instances where they know they need help). In addition, the uneven nature of demand in maternity assures the periodic availability of time for nurses to do the coding work. Finally, since almost none of these patients is covered by Medicare, in some states it may not matter much if we get the code right anyway.

General medical patients. It takes eighty or more DRGs to encompass the vast majority of their conditions. The clinical differences can be quite subtle but can also have profound reimbursement implications. Furthermore, the majority of these patients are covered by Medicare. Getting the coding right is a key factor on the revenue line for this portion of our business.

Within the traditional operating structure of most hospitals today, both of these sets of patient charts are handled in exactly the same way; they go to a black hole, stay there awhile, are assembled, and are finally coded by a nonmedical worker. Even without radical changes, this process could be improved. For many hospitals, it would be appropriate for the obstetrics (OB) nursing staff to code their own records in their spare time. To code medical patients' records, it may be appropriate to undertake a national search and pay $75,000 a year to retain the services of the best "medicine coder" in the country. Currently, we overserve OB and underserve general medicine.

Similar examples could easily fill a separate volume. In fact, hospitalwide restructuring is a search for all the significant instances of service and cost imbalances and the attempt to redress them systematically for defined sets of patients. Taking this larger and more comprehensive view is critical to the process because we would find ourselves unable to solve most problems in an isolated manner. Let us return to the housekeeping example. It might be very tempting to close the book at this point, go to the office tomorrow, and attempt to redeploy housekeepers to the various nursing units. Unfortunately, we would quickly discover that there are not enough to go around. We are then faced with two equally unattractive choices—reduce service levels or add housekeepers (in other words, cost)—neither of which addresses the goal we had in mind. The problem arises from the combination of two factors; it is created not only by the inefficiencies of centralization but also by the narrow job focus of the housekeepers themselves. If we merely decentralize or redeploy, we do nothing to fix the other major source of structural idle time. Only by involving a larger pool of functions in the restructuring framework will we be able to extract the hidden value.

The Domination of Routine Work

There is a perception in the general public and even within our field that much of the work of the modern hospital is dominated by rocket science—taking bullets out of brains, removing steering wheels from chests, inserting scopes where God never intended, taking pictures of subcellular chemical processes, and transplanting an increasingly impressive array of organs. Yes, we do these things and do them in growing numbers. But the truth of the matter is that the majority of all nonnursing transactions in the hospital are simpler and more routine tests and procedures. For example, between 50 and 60 percent of all inpatient general radiology procedures are chest X rays. Add in abdominal series and extremity films, and the number is even higher. Special studies, MRIs, and CAT scans are a fairly small percentage of the total number of procedures demanded (although their high cost tends to warp our perception of their volume and overall contribution to work load).

Table 4.1 depicts a typical profile of the most common procedures and tests and their cumulative contribution to total, nonnursing transactions. The procedures included add up to a total of about thirty or so line items: high-volume, automated chemistries (mostly electrolytes); basic hematology work-ups; chest, abdominal, and extremity films; basic respiratory care (not ventilators); and basic EKG services. Together, these thirty items account for 65 to 80 percent of all the demand for centralized ancillary services. These ranges are typical and tend to be as true of academic medical centers as they are of 200-bed community hospitals.

This emerging profile of the hospital's work load departs even further from conventional wisdom when we discover that

Table 4.1. Concentration of Routine Services.

Service Type	Cumulative Percentage of Total Nonnursing Transactions
Basic hematology	26%
Basic chemistry	46%
Chest-extremity films	57%
Basic respiratory	64%
EKG	68%

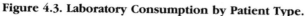

Figure 4.3. Laboratory Consumption by Patient Type.

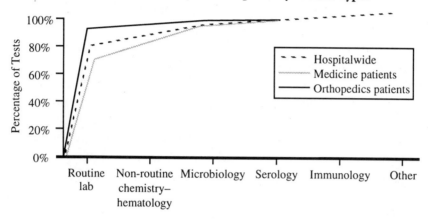

it does not much matter whether we are looking at open-heart patients or ear, nose, and throat (ENT) patients. The dominance of routine procedures still pertains. Yes, an open-heart surgery may get fifty of these common items in a twenty-four-hour period, whereas an ENT patient requires only five or six. Yet in each case, they account for a remarkably similar percentage of each patient's ancillary requirements, as shown in Figure 4.3.

Implications

This somewhat surprising information can be very good news indeed to those seeking to reduce costs and improve performance. It tells us that we do not have to fix everything to have a significant impact on service to patients and physicians and on our cost of doing business. If we can focus on these thirty or so high-volume, relatively straightforward procedures and tests, we can affect 70 percent or more of all the nonnursing clinical transactions of our patients—hospitalwide. But the opportunity will not be realized simply by making the lab or radiology more "productive" since those specific components of the processes are only small fractions of the overall complexity and flow of tests and films. An all-encompassing view of the work involved, its patterns of demand, and the intricate connections to other steps in the care process will be needed.

The other important implication is that this new understanding of the volume and concentration of overall transactions liberates us to explore entirely new avenues of thought, to open up previously unthinkable solutions. This is a classic example of how paradigms work and change. The new paradigm solves a problem that under the old system was deemed hopeless. In the old world, a common service problem in radiology (such as complaints about waiting time) would likely be addressed as follows:

- The CEO or a vice president would mobilize a task force consisting of nurses, the radiology staff, ward clerks, and perhaps transporters.
- After three months of diligent study, the task force would submit its conclusions and recommendations. It might find that there are not enough transporters, a shortage that causes patients to wait to be taken to X ray and to be returned to their rooms following their procedures.
- The CEO acts on the recommendation and hires several more transporters.
- After six months, there is no dramatic reduction in the stream of complaints. The CEO reactivates the task force. The task force studies the problem for another three months.
- Its new report, delivered a bit sheepishly, says that now that the hospital has enough transporters for radiology, the true, underlying problem with radiology waiting times has been unmasked. The hospital does not have enough elevators!

Now, before the CEO (or you, gentle reader) runs out and authorizes two new elevator shafts at $250,000 each, think about what we have learned about radiology demand by inpatients. Stop and imagine a world where 60 percent of the patients currently riding elevators up and down to radiology did not have to ride elevators at all. Think of the work that goes away if we can provide chest films on the patient care floors. We could eliminate

- Scheduling transactions and multiple phone calls
- Transporting the patient to radiology and back again
- Multiple log-in–log-out and handoff transactions

Just as importantly, the patient is not inconvenienced by two trips through public areas or subjected to waiting in radiology before and after the procedure. In addition, the patient is not rendered unavailable for other procedures for the two or more hours that centralized X rays can now require. And finally, a substantial load on hospital elevators can be eliminated, improving service for visitors, physicians, staff members, and patients requiring more sophisticated procedures.

As fascinating as this opportunity is, remember that this one idea alone will not solve all our problems. In and of itself, it will save a few minutes a day for each ward clerk in the hospital, save some time for the radiology schedulers, and probably reduce the demand for transportation services. But if we are going to realize this gain, we will have to combine it with other opportunities and restructure large parts of the total work involved in patient care. This conclusion brings us directly to the next part of our story, the relative absence of true "economies of scale" in a service business with highly changeable demand.

Scale Versus Utilization Effects

It is taken as an article of faith that economies of scale exist in every business endeavor and that it is part of the job of management to seek out such opportunities and capitalize on them. In its most basic form, this axiom can be stated as the more units of x that one produces, the lower the cost per unit. It is a very sensible attitude, and dramatic examples abound: for example, if we do 100,000 pounds of laundry in a given set of machines, it will cost less per pound than doing only 75,000 pounds of laundry with the same machines. We will not have to hire additional managers or purchase additional machines to handle the increased volume. We may not even have to hire additional staff if the machines themselves handle the bulk of the work involved.

But the story is more complicated than this. True, if we use the machines at higher percentages of their capacities, we win—especially if the machines' work steps constitute the bulk of the work involved. The acid test when applying this concept to a given business or activity is to assess whether throughput is optimal (or at least predictable) and whether the process in question dominates the overall work load. Let us see how this applies in the hospital.

Consider a common management decision in the hospital: the economics of acquiring a bigger or faster multichannel chemistry analyzer for the laboratory. For our purposes here, we will call it the WhizBang 2000. The selling features of the WhizBang 2000 are as follows:

- It can process fifty samples per hour, a significant improvement over our current machine (the CrummyChem 100, which handles only thirty samples per hour).
- The WhizBang 2000 is very stingy with reagents and will reduce our reagent cost per test from $.10 to $.08.

On the surface, the WhizBang 2000 appears to offer scale economies and speed, as well as technology-enabled reagent savings. The decision is obvious: throw out the CrummyChem and install the WhizBang. Yet before we send our check to the manufacturer, we should look at demand for chemistry tests and see what we are really buying for our money in terms of service and cost. Figure 4.4 presents a typical but schematic view of demand for automated chemistry tests (routine, not stat) by hour of the day.

Given the way most laboratories set up their service schedules, we should not be surprised to see the peaks in demand—the steepest peak in the early morning and a second, much smaller

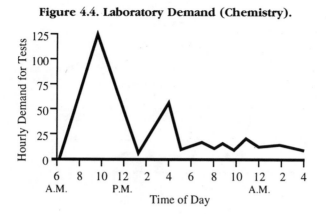

Figure 4.4. Laboratory Demand (Chemistry).

peak in the early afternoon. What happens in between can almost be described as random noise in the system: very small batches. This assessmemt is borne out when we look at the frequency distribution of batch sizes in the chemistry lab, which often shows that the majority of batches consist of fewer than three specimens.

One laboratory director once used these curves to explain why he needed to staff for peak demand in the lab: "We're like a fire department; we have to be ready to respond." However, given that the lab generally mandates its own service schedules that result in the peaks of demand, it might be more accurate to describe the lab as a fire department that upon reporting to work proceeds to set a very large fire—the better to make sure that it will be busy! While daily rounds and acquired patterns of attending physicians certainly play a role in determining the demand curve for laboratory services, the situation is not completely different from the need to change all patients' beds in the morning because that is when the housekeepers have structured their operations to do the work.

But to return to the main line of our story, what does this demand curve tell us about the potential efficacy of the WhizBang 2000? Figure 4.5 adds the hourly throughput of the WhizBang 2000 to the earlier chemistry demand curve. Suddenly, the new machine does not appear to be the miracle that was advertised.

Figure 4.5. Laboratory Demand (Chemistry) with Hourly Throughput.

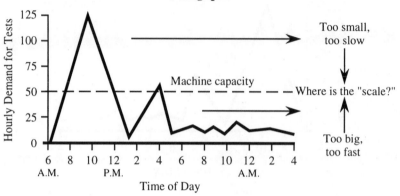

What the graph reveals is that the WhizBang 2000 is woefully inadequate to the task at hand during the two-hour morning peak. Its throughput of fifty specimens per hour is only about one-third the capacity we need. Worse than that, for up to twenty hours per day, this latest marvel is five to ten times as fast and as big as we need. Where is the economy of scale? To the extent that such economies exist, they are dwarfed by countervailing utilization penalties. The volume and pattern of demand simply prevent us from extracting much, if any, of the theoretical scale effects. The WhizBang 2000 (or perhaps several of them) would be most useful in a large, commercial reference laboratory whose demand curve is quite conveniently smoothed by the luxury of very large batches and relatively long turnaround time (usually twenty-four hours).

In a hospital with predictable peaks in demand, the scale effects are erased by the fact that the machine probably has the same number of assigned staff members on any given shift regardless of the number of samples being put through the device. Furthermore, the entire support infrastructure to feed the machine is also in place—whether two samples are being processed or fifty. All the ward clerks, phlebotomists, accessioning clerks, lab supervisors, and pathologists remain on duty throughout a given shift. These costs dwarf the direct machine-based costs of the test itself. It is helpful to review the process flow chart for a typical lab test, noting particularly the small number of steps actually represented by the performance of the test.

Why would we then buy the WhizBang 2000? Two reasons are possible. First, the savings on reagents could add up to several thousand dollars per year, and this benefit should not be ignored. At the same time, before taking this finding at face value, a bit of homework on actual reagent use to keep the machine constantly ready would be needed. Does the machine actually consume no reagents to be in a ready state? Does the cleaning and calibration process use a fixed amount of reagents regardless of the number of tests run during the preceding period? If so, the actual per-specimen costs will be affected. It might also be worthwhile to see if the hospital will actually order enough reagents during the year to get the anticipated volume discount. The second benefit is faster processing of the day's peak of demand. The WhizBang 2000 will indeed plow through the morning rush more quickly than the CrummyChem 100. As we will see, though, this peak could perhaps be smoothed by a more responsive operating approach that does not compress all that demand into one two-hour window in the first place—thus eliminating the need for the very advantage the WhizBang 2000 hopes to deliver.

The laboratory example of scale versus utilization can be reproduced in almost any department or function in the hospital. It is very much like the faulty concept of traditional productivity that we discussed in relation to the admitting office and other activities. Perhaps the common thread is the parallel between notions of "scale" and "productivity." What our current paradigm obscures from us is that both notions assume a given operational approach and work only within that structure. Our clue to this insight is the word *scale* itself. It should alert us to the fact that we are working and thinking within a defined, calibrated space. This decision is fine in a sense, but it confines our thinking and dictates the metrics of productivity that are appropriate to the chosen operating approach. Restructuring is about redefining the scale itself. When we do this, it makes it very easy to see that today's "emperor of productivity" is often wearing no clothes.

Misguided Demand-Side Initiatives

Just as the demand side can point us in the right direction and focus our energies on significant opportunities, it can also help us move away from areas of limited potential. Reducing the consumption of ancillary services by inpatients is a common strategy that hospitals use to address payers' concerns, as well as a means of reducing institutional costs. There may indeed be reasons to attack ancillary consumption, but improved financial performance is not one of them. We can return to the laboratory and see why this is so.

Let us say that a hospital of five hundred beds has embarked on an aggressive effort to reduce the number of lab tests ordered for inpatients (presumably by eliminating marginal or redundant utilization). Let us further assume that the effort succeeds wildly; the consumption of lab tests is reduced by one full test per patient per day. At 80 percent occupancy, this means that there are four hundred fewer inpatient lab tests ordered per day. What will this figure produce?

- In terms of gross revenue, the hospital has reduced its top line by $8,000 per day (using $20 as the average charge per test).
- The effect on net revenue will depend on the percentage of hospital revenue that is accounted for by fixed payment schemes (Medicare DRGs, for instance) and the bad-debt rate. Unless the hospital is operated by a prepaid healthcare plan, it is likely that at least 20 to 40 percent of the gross revenue will get translated into net revenue by charge-based payers. In other words, the reduction in lab orders translates directly into $1,600 to $3,200 of lost net revenue—real cash money.
- The effect on the cost side (to compensate for the lost net revenue) is much harder to identify with any certainty. For

openers, we can optimistically estimate that the hospital might save $.50 per test on reagents and supplies—a total of $200 per day. That leaves a gap of $1,400 to $3,000 to close between lost net revenue and direct savings on reagents and supplies. At $15 per hour per technologist, we would have to reduce the staff in the laboratory by about twelve to twenty-five FTEs in order to close the gap fully.

Unfortunately, the probability of cutting the staff by even one FTE is by no means high. Though four hundred fewer tests per day sounds significant, by the time the difference is spread out across three shifts and across most sections of the clinical lab, the impact on individual work loads gets highly diluted. Furthermore, the impact on the test-ordering infrastructure is even more diminished. In effect, this is a losing proposition for the institution. It also illustrates the notion discussed earlier: it is almost impossible to chase the volume curve down with the cost curve. Revenue goes down at the average, whereas costs go down at the margin.

Of course, there are good reasons to reduce the consumption of ancillary services. The primary one ought to be that patients are inconvenienced unnecessarily (stuck with needles, rolled through the halls, and so forth) and in some cases even compromised clinically (too much radiation exposure). Further, in the long run, we can use the reduced consumption levels to rescale the operational approach and to develop multidisciplinary protocols for certain types of patients. Regrettably, most hospital consumption-reduction initiatives are merely doomed efforts targeted at relatively near-term improvements in financial performance and driven by an incomplete view of the limitations of the current operating structure.

A Source of Scale—or at Least Synergy

We need not despair completely of finding leverage in size. There are many areas of the hospital where greater volume or larger size leads to savings. Perhaps the most important example for our purposes here is in nursing-unit size. The benefits of increasing the size of nursing units are not wholly related to scale, but they are significant and give us another leverage point to exploit as we restructure hospital operations.

There are two key advantages to increasing the size of nursing units: reduced variation in the hours of care delivered to patients and reduced management overhead. We will leave aside for the moment how we decide which patients can be appropriately and effectively aggregated into these larger units; that will be the subject of a separate chapter. Here we want to understand the nature of the advantages that exist if we can succeed in managing larger groupings of patients.

Let us look first at the coverage and hours-of-care dimension. Figure 4.6 shows the number of beds, staffing, and average daily census for two relatively small but typical nursing units. The more interesting data is to be found in the demand patterns for each unit. Unit *A* had three days during the month when the patient census exceeded the planned staffing capacity, and Unit *B* also had three days, for a total of six days between the two units. These overcapacity days result in one or both of two undesirable outcomes. Either the unit squeaks by with its normal staffing (presumably paying some service penalty in the process), or the unit acquires additional resources (staff members) from somewhere else—either transferred temporarily from another unit, retained from an agency, given overtime, or some combination of these

Figure 4.6. Demand on Two Small Units.

Unit A	Unit B
Patient census = 32 Staff members = 50 Days understaffed = 3	Patient census = 17 Staff members = 25 Days understaffed = 3

Figure 4.7. "Law of Large Numbers."

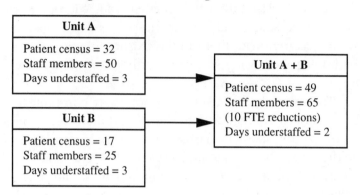

factors. In either event, we have paid a penalty in terms of customer service or cost (or both).

Let us see, however, what happens when we use these same patient demand patterns but roll them up into a larger entity. Figure 4.7 shows what happens if we combine Units *A* and *B*. In common sense terms, the law of large numbers asserts itself to our advantage. Fewer staff are capable of meeting demand more often on the combined unit; a staff of sixty-five results in only two days when demand exceeds planned staffing capacity. To make this perhaps surprising outcome more transparent, we should consider two somewhat extreme examples. If we have a unit with a staffed census target of just three patients, we are in real trouble if we ever get four patients on the unit. We have experienced a 33 percent increase in demand. By contrast, if we have a unit staffed for a census of fifty patients and we actually have fifty-one patients, we have only experienced a 2 percent increase in work load. The smaller work load increase is obviously easier to absorb. On the demand side of the situation, we also benefit. There is a greater possibility that variations in census will smooth out when a larger universe of patients is in play. In this way, the law of large numbers assists us in meeting patient needs more consistently with a smaller staff. Without worrying about *how* we select patients for these larger aggregations (or how we accommodate them in the existing physical structure), the advantages of doing so makes further consideration worthwhile.

The example just given does not really constitute a scale effect; it derives from utilization. The other dimension of the issue of nursing unit size—management infrastructure—is a classic scale-driven effect. Nursing units have fairly predictable management arrangements—at least a minimum of these, although many hospitals have more layers, specialists, and coordinators than discussed here. A nursing unit of thirty or so beds will usually have a head nurse on at least two of the three standard shifts. In addition, we are likely to find a charge nurse structure below that level and a piece of a "director" at the next level up. We know this structure does not represent the maximum span of control that is possible because we will find almost the same management arrangements for units ranging in size from twenty beds up to forty beds or more. Further, clerical support is also dependent on the number of units the hospital has as well as the clerical load specific to unit size (that is, we need at least one clerk no matter how small the unit). Above that level, clerks are added based on work load and coverage requirements.

If we combine these two effects—the law of large numbers and management scale—we can construct a somewhat crude scale curve for nursing unit size, as shown in Figure 4.8.

The important features of the curve are that there is a strong overall scale effect and that the rate of increased benefits decays substantially above unit sizes of about one hundred beds. In fact, the majority of the benefits are realized at about sixty or seventy beds. This finding means that we should strive to create larger aggregations of patients; at the same time, we must realize that pushing this idea to its theoretical limit will involve chasing incrementally smaller improvements.

Before we leave this topic, a subtle but important point

Figure 4.8. Impact of Larger Nursing Units.

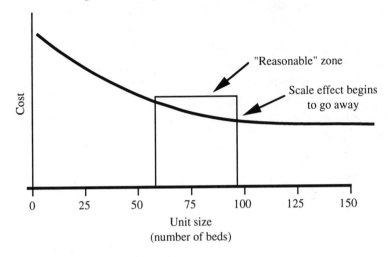

should be noted. This curve was constructed using today's operating structure and economics. This illustration is very useful in pointing us in a different direction for the future, but it can also be deceptive. When we eventually restructure the operation, a different set of economics will apply to the analysis. As we will see later, the new operating structure will present us with new challenges for optimizing the performance of a unit of any given size—even as we strive where possible to increase the size of units. As we move more direct staff members to the units, smaller unit sizes will not be a problem in the same way they are now. When smaller units are necessary, they will challenge us to use unit-based specialists (for example, radiology technologists) productively, perhaps across an array of functions and tasks.

It is clear at this point in our journey that the present operating structure of hospitals is deeply flawed. Whether we view the hospital from the supply side or the demand side of the issue, we find profound discontinuities and processes hopelessly out of proportion to their roles in the clinical care of patients. Service levels to our key customers—patients and physicians—have deteriorated to the point that it is almost a miracle that they put up with them. Technology enhancements are seldom translated into service benefits. Most troubling is the fact that our efforts to make improvements have been condemned to failure by the limitations of our vision and our unwillingness to let go of our traditional operating paradigm. But we now have enough evidence to strike out in a new direction. We know what the problems are, and it is now time to identify the nature and imperatives of a new operating structure for future hospitals—one that focuses on patients.

5

The Structure

of a New

Paradigm

Hospitals are not going to solve their operational problems by implementing incremental changes. By and large, we have spent the last three decades in a vain attempt to influence operating performance through such mechanisms. Our failures as an industry can be read in the inexorable year-to-year increases in the hospital–medical care portion of the consumer price index. Although we are not without some small victories and can resort to a list of mitigating factors (technology, intensity of care, population aging, defensive medicine), the fact remains that it is nearly impossible to point to any specific initiatives that have sustainably reduced overall costs. Group purchasing and price bashing of manufacturers have slowed the growth of supply costs, but lasting changes in employee head counts per occupied bed have not occurred. Furthermore, guest relations programs may have succeeded in achieving marginal gains in the quality of face-to-face interactions with customers, but unwieldy processes have not been simplified or streamlined. Improvements in customer service have amounted to little more than providing smiling faces for patients to see as they wend their way through the mazes that hospitals have designed to accomplish relatively straightforward tasks. Until the structure changes, such superficial efforts will continue to dominate the landscape.

This chapter presents a high-level, structural view of the future of hospital operations—a glimpse of a new paradigm. Rather than attempting to deduce this new paradigm, we will simply invoke one capable of addressing the problems dealt with so far. By making estimates of what is possible, we will propose a new value-added structure for the hospital of the future. Let us remind ourselves of our goals.

- Improve continuity of care for our patients
- Improve the continuity of professional relationships among care givers and doctors as they collaborate on behalf of patients
- Minimize the movement of patients through the hospital
- Increase the proportion of direct-care activities when compared to infrastructure work
- Tailor operating environments to the particular needs of related groups of patients
- Empower staff members to plan and execute their work in ways that are most responsive to patient needs

Using these goals and reassessing the old value-added structure, we can postulate the general shape of a new model. By making estimates of the potential improvements in various value-added components, we have derived a new general structure, shown in Figure 5.1. First, medical-technical-clinical care *is* our business, and we should devote as much of our resources to it as possible. These are the activities that are obvious to our customers and are therefore those from which our staffs derive the greatest satisfaction. The new value-added structure suggests that 24 percent of our efforts—the largest single component by far—be directly devoted to patient health care. Despite overall

Figure 5.1. Value-Added Structures.

	Today	Vision
	$1.00	
Medical–technical –clinical services	$.16–16%	$.70–$.80
Hotel services	$.08–8%	$.24–30%
Medical documentation	$.19–19%	$.11–14%
Institutional documentation	$.11–11%	$.10–13%
Scheduling–coordination	$.14–14%	$.08–11%
Transportation	$.06–6%	$.04–6%
Management and supervision	$.07–7%	$.06–8%
Ready for action time	$.19–19%	$.06–8%
		$.08–10%

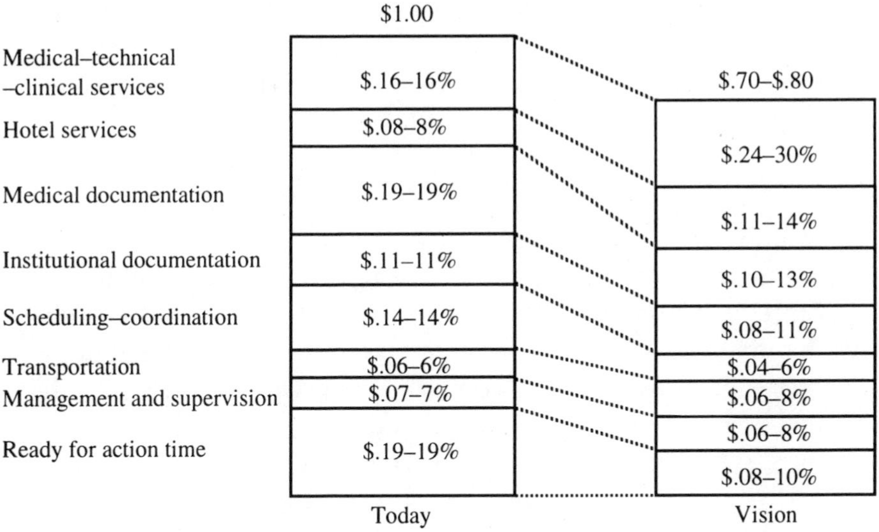

costs that are projected to be lower than today, the absolute resources devoted to these activities would increase. In other
words, we would do everything for patients that we do today but
do it better—with substantial increases in direct contacts. Most
of these gains will be along the cognitive dimension of patient
care: planning, counseling, comforting, and educating.

The second thing to understand about the two value-added
structures is that we will not get from today to tomorrow by
working harder and faster. We will only get there by eliminating—structurally—the need to do a lot of the unnecessary and
minimally valuable work that the operating structure now requires. Transporting X ray patients at full gallop will not improve
continuity of care, reduce structural idle time, enhance turnaround time, or save any money. Eliminating the need for off-
unit transports for basic X rays will let us make progress in all
those areas. Performing today's work more quickly is only likely
to result in higher levels of structural idle time—since our history
of being able to realize such paper gains in productivity is dismal

indeed. Similarly, writing faster (or typing on computers faster) will not significantly affect the paperwork burden. Using multidisciplinary protocols and only charting exceptions (for patient types where this is possible) will produce a step-change improvement in documentation time.

The Importance of Ends, Not Means

At this point, it might seem that what it is being advocated is merely massive cross training and moving ancillary equipment onto the patient floors. Well, yes and no. Those are indeed two important means. But the ends are far more important and must be reemphasized to avoid confusing the particular situation with the overriding principles that guide us.

The principle at work here was developed very early—probably at the third or fourth meeting with the original six-client consortium some five years ago. When the analysis was presented to the group (the hospitals' senior executives), they were asked, "Did you know that fifty to sixty employees interact with a patient who stays an average of four-days at your hospitals?" The senior nurse executives said they suspected that the number was big but had no idea that it was that large. They agreed that involving that many individuals in the care of a typical general surgery patient certainly constituted bad service and almost certainly constituted bad care as well. They asked if an operating structure could be designed that would produce the following result: for most patients, on most shifts, the hospital staff would consist of two or three faces.

The answer to this challenge is, of course, that it *is* feasible. Hospital operations can be designed so that most patients need only deal with two or three staff members per shift for most of their care. If this is to be done, however, two key changes must be accomplished. First, the parade of those performing narrow tasks must be eliminated from the patient's room. Second, the necessity of patients meeting three or four strangers in the course of receiving a routine service from a centralized ancillary department must be removed.

To accomplish these objectives, we will have to train our staff so that fewer people perform a broader range of functions for smaller groups of patients—thus reducing the number of individuals the patient must encounter to get basic care. We will also have to investigate the feasibility of moving high-volume ancillary procedures to the patient floors; this approach would decrease the need for the patient to meet transporters, receptionists, and clerks in centralized departments. Whether we can also train nursing staffs to perform basic X rays and lab work (or train X ray and lab technicians to perform many routine bedside-care tasks) will depend on the laws of the state, the patient population to be served, unit size, and institutional preferences and realities.

Nevertheless, the end we seek is greater continuity of care and improved service (with reduced cost in the bargain), not cross training or equipment redeployment for their own sakes. Those are simply two of the most likely means of achieving our goals.

A Changing Paradigm of "Ownership"

Ownership is an underlying imperative of the new paradigm. In fact, our very notion of ownership must change. In the current compartmentalized operating structure, ownership is fragmented at best. Since no one in the organization is responsible for a broad set of patient care activities, *ownership* is narrowly defined as relating to a limited set of tasks ("I must fill 130 prescriptions today") or area of the hospital ("I'm responsible for Exam Room 3"). Ultimate accountability to the customer is nearly impossible. We can see countless examples of this problem in our daily work—or at least we *could* see countless examples if we were to view the world from a new set of optics.

Consider the strange behavior that takes place throughout our organizations, behavior that would be unthinkable if the notion of ownership changed from departments and tasks to patients. Let us look at an example from the operating rooms. On an average day in many hospitals, we can make the following predictions about the status of the work force in the operating rooms at about 2:00 P.M.:

- The holding and prep areas will have no patients but will still be staffed (at least partially).
- About one-half—perhaps more—of the operating rooms will be empty. However, the staffs of at least some of these rooms will be on duty until 3:00 P.M. or so.
- The recovery room will be the busiest of the three areas, but it is still likely that not all staff members will be fully utilized late in the afternoon.
- Although some members of the staff may be performing cleaning tasks or preparing for the next day's setup and schedule, others are simply idle—ready for action.

The inefficiency of this staff utilization model is striking. Yet the more important issue here is ownership and the way it currently manifests itself. Why does it never occur to any of the operating room staff members to do something with this structural idle time that would add value to patients? The opportunities to do so are staring them (and us) in the face.

- Circulating nurses (or some of them, at least) could perhaps stay with their last patients of the day in the recovery room. This practice would be aimed not at reducing the staffing level in the recovery room but at improving the staff's understanding of the entire care process, even if only within one functional area.
- On other occasions, circulating nurses might visit one or two of their day's patients back on the surgical nursing unit. These visits would "close the loop" on two integrally related pieces of the care process for surgical patients. In the process, the circulating nurses might learn something valuable about the postoperative consequences of various surgical procedures, options, and techniques.

- Recovery room nurses might occasionally transport their final patient of the day back to the nursing unit and check up on the progress of one or two of their patients from earlier in the day. The idea is not to eliminate any transporters; it is another effort to instill a broader sense of ownership.

Of course, our structural paradigm would not need to change to permit the behaviors just suggested; we could begin encouraging staff members to do these things today. But we should not confuse cause and effect and blame our people for acting as they do. Today's compartmentalized behaviors did not create our operating structure; our operating structure encouraged our staffs to become compartmentalized. The sad part of this situation is not just that our ability to provide more compassionate and personal care has been compromised. The real tragedy may be that our staff members are robbed of opportunities to feel that they are integral parts of a larger process. How do we instill a sense of ownership in pharmacists, for instance, who work in a central dispensary and may never come in contact with a single patient? How will a radiology technician understand patients' broader needs and concerns when the work day consists of a series of ten-minute, assembly-line transactions with patients who may never return to the department? How will a food service worker who delivers carts to floors (but not trays to patients) ever appreciate the importance of food in the daily lives of patients or judge whether or not hospital food and service are adequate? Even compassionate and caring employees can be forgiven for their tunnel vision when we understand that the structure virtually requires this point of view—especially when we hold our people to "production standards" that are purely departmental.

In any structure we wish to devise, even managers will have structural idle time (in addition to the considerable amounts of discretionary time inherent in management duties). Much has been written about "management by walking around," especially in manufacturing settings. In service businesses (especially hospitals), we can suggest a further refinement: "management by making something better" for a patient or a family member. Opportunities to make things better for our customers are not hard to find. We can spontaneously visit the waiting room in the emergency department. We can offer to call a cab for a patient and pay for it (the $20 will not affect this quarter's profit or loss). We can ask the dietary department to bring a coffee and soft drink cart for those waiting (the cafeteria will never miss the revenue). Since waiting is one of the chief activities of our customers, it would be many months before we would run out of areas to visit. The impact on patients would be considerable and the example we set for our employees would probably be contagious.

Ownership and Empowerment: Two Examples

Empowerment is inherent in any notion of ownership. If employees do not have the skills, discretion, incentive, and structure that enable ownership of patients, nothing much will change. Ownership begins with a clear sense of goals—an understanding of what business we are in, what is important, and where each activity fits in. As a bit of relief from theory and numbers, we can humanize these concepts with two real-world examples of empowerment and ownership.

The first story concerns an activity that management typically considers a perennial problem and a source of some discretionary revenue: parking. Anyone who has ever had the misfortune of trying to exit a hospital parking structure around the time of shift change will know the difficulty that arises when lots of cars try to get through the bottleneck: the toll booth. The problem is compounded almost exponentially for those on the top of a multilevel structure. From recent personal experience, it is no exaggeration to say that the process can take an hour or more. As we sit in line, slowly wending our way down the ramps, we should take the opportunity to think about what is going on from a customer service point of view—particularly in relation to empowerment and ownership. Let us consider the employee in the toll booth.

What we might like that employee to be thinking is, The $75 I'm going to collect in the next hour is not worth the aggravation caused by the long wait our customers will have to endure. The bad will created more than outweighs the money. Heck, we're not in the parking business, we're in the patient care business. We might also hope that as a result of this brilliant insight, the toll-booth employee would raise the gate, wave all the cars through, and smile at each driver. Unfortunately, however, that employee probably has a quite different reaction. He or she is probably thinking, Business is *great*! Every time I look up, there's another customer waiting to give me money!

Now before we get mad at the toll-booth employee, we need to remind ourselves that the operating structure of the 1990s virtually precludes the kind of thinking that would inspire opening the gate. The structure tells the employee that hospitals *are* in the parking business. Moreover, a true visionary occupying that position who in fact opened the gate and let everyone out for free would certainly be fired! The insight about not being in the parking business (ownership) is necessary but not sufficient. The action of opening the gate without the risk of getting fired (empowerment) must also be encouraged by the culture and values of the organization.

If the parking lot story represents an example of what is currently wrong, the following anecdote describes what we should strive for. It involves the first day of operations after a forty-bed orthopedics unit is converted to the pardigm of patient-focused care. At this particular hospital, the new model includes a minilab on the floor, staffed more or less full time by a medical technologist who is considered part of the overall patient care team for the unit. Around 10:00 A.M. on this anxiety-filled day, one of the nurses approaches the vice president who is responsible for the conversion (and who has therefore virtually lived on the floor around the clock for several days).

The nurse was confused by a lab report she had received from the new minilab on the floor. Its results looked just like those she had received for the same tests run by the central lab the prior evening (just before the conversion of the unit). She did not understand why this report needed to be generated again by the new minilab. The vice president was at a loss to explain the situation, so she suggested they visit the minilab together to get to the bottom of things. The laboratory technician in the mini-lab was very helpful. He carefully looked up the report in his log for the day. The answer was easy, "Oh, those are the results for those same tests that were ordered again for that patient this morning." The nurse was amazed, "But I just drew that sample an hour ago!"

But that is not the punch line of the story. The lab technician then very calmly and sincerely added, "That's all right; we'll get better." Imagine the probability of that exchange taking place today. Here is a lab technician who understands what business the hospital is really in (patient care) and his place in that business. He is close enough to patients to feel an obligation directly to them, as well as to other team members involved in their care. Furthermore, the new structure (particularly the redeployment of the lab equipment) empowers him to act on his new understanding.

A New Management Paradigm

It is not just the staff members at the bedside for whom *ownership* and *empowerment* should take on new meaning. Our entire conception of hospital organization structures must be transformed. If we do not change our management arrangements to fit the new order, our other efforts will fail. If the manager of the parking operation described earlier is not attuned to the new paradigm, the toll-booth attendant who allows the cars to exit free of charge will still get fired.

We can begin by looking once again at how we currently organize our management teams. But before we look at a single organizational chart, we should take an even higher-level view of what we are trying to manage—to see the product and short-

Table 5.1. Today's Resource Allocation.

Administration (15%)	
Numerous Clerical and Administrative Activities	
Ancillary (25%)	*Nursing* (40%)
Diagnostic, therapeutic, and invasive procedures	Routine and specialized nursing care
Support (20%)	
General patient support and facility-related services	

comings of today's paradigm. Table 5.1 provides a somewhat unusual view of the current organization. It looks at where resources are grouped and managed, as well as their relative amounts.

The first number that should be noted is the surprisingly small percentage of resources deployed and managed more or less at the bedside. This category includes only nursing care and amounts to just 30 to 40 percent of our total personnel resources (depending on how we count nursing management and related overhead). All the other resources needed by patients are provided by other centralized departments. Management of patient care therefore becomes a hopelessly tangled matrix of functions and relationships. Previous chapters have dealt with this dimension of the problem at some length.

A more subtle outgrowth of this structure is the impediment it presents to intelligent decision making. This sort of structure creates two important problems: it forces management decision making to the highest levels of the organization, and it often leads us to make less-than-astute decisions. To the first point, we only need to consider what needs to happen in order to answer a relatively straightforward question: "How's the cardiac surgery business doing?" Hardly any individual below the CEO is in a position to answer this question fully. The head nurses involved may know that census is up (but may not know that longer length of stay is creating that increase) and that there are two vacant positions on weekends. The operating room supervisor may recognize that both surgeries and surgical hours per procedure have increased. The CFO may be worried that the payer mix is deteriorating. Respiratory therapists may see that the consumption of procedures (say, ventilator care and arterial blood gases) has declined on a per-stay basis. The pharmacy may know that a new drug may ultimately reduce the need to perform open-heart surgery. And medical records personnel may recognize that Doctor M's length of stay and postsurgical complications are outside of predicted norms and peer results.

Many people know important information about cardiac surgery at the hospital. Unfortunately, the structure conspires against anyone who wishes to take a broad view of the service. In most cases, the CEO is left to figure out who should be asked what and how the pieces should be put together to get a general picture of the cardiac surgery business. Some hospitals have product-line managers to perform this tedious matrixing activity; however, because these are usually staff positions, the individuals holding them are nearly powerless to do anything with the answers. In fact, the very term *product-line management* is misleading because there are no "line" reporting relationships involved. Perhaps we should retitle such individuals as "product-line matrixers."

Another problem arises in a business where only 30 or 40 percent of the costs are direct (in this case, managed at the bedside). Decision making (especially financial decision making) is cumbersome and fraught with pitfalls for the unwary. Let us illustrate this problem with a real-life example from a community hospital in the Northwest. The market of this hospital is dominated by managed care—upwards of 80 percent of clients not covered by Medicare and Medicaid have HMO-type insurance. The hospitals get reimbursement through various per-diem and discount arrangements.

The staff at the hospital was concerned about the impact of the HMOs on its maternity business. Eighty-five percent of unit patients were covered by an HMO, and most of those plans required that normal deliveries be discharged within twenty-four hours. From a customer-service perspective, this was an obvious problem. The new mothers were tired and sore and had no desire to go back to the rigors of normal home life within one day—especially those mothers with other children at home. An extra day or two of what amounted to very low-intensity, respite care would have been welcomed by the majority of the OB patients (almost all of whom could be described as middle class and had the resources to pay for some discretionary services). Furthermore, census on the unit averaged only about 55 percent.

The staff thus considered developing a program that would let such patients stay extra nights for a nominal charge (about the same, say, as a night at a Holiday Inn). What stood in the way of this customer-responsive innovation? Well, the CFO ran the hospital's light-dimming computer model that allocated costs to the OB unit. On a fully loaded basis, it cost over $600 to keep a maternity patient overnight. The staff was stymied and did not implement a program that might in the long run have drawn additional deliveries to the hospital.

Such decisions fly in the face of common sense. The unit would not have added any staff members to care for these essentially "well" patients. The hospital would not have had to feed them more food than that discarded as a rounding error from the kitchen on any given day. The hospital *would* have had $75 or $100 in its pocket for each additional day of stay. The hospital would have also had happier customers who might have passed on the word to their friends.

Why was the plan impossible? Over the years, the operating structure has forced management to make decisions like this—using allocated costs as the basis. The problem with this approach is that decisions are based on information about averages, when most decisions about existing programs are played out at the margin. While we receive "average" revenue for any given service, we only incur "marginal" costs. This makes management difficult, because we tend to think in terms of averages (costs, revenues, and so forth). This leads to bad decisions. The OB situation provides a perfect example: common sense tells us the incremental (marginal) costs are negligible and the revenues (cash we can count) are easily identified. There is no need to look any further, and any examination of allocated costs is unnecessary.

To use an analogy from another industry: McDonald's would never have gotten into the breakfast business if it had analyzed fully allocated costs. Low-revenue breakfast items would have appeared to lose money for the company and its stores. But McDonald's executives knew that taxes, rent, utilities, insurance, and most other infrastructure costs would not be significantly affected. They probably just looked at the extra revenue and the new direct costs (raw food and wages). There is little chance that they regret the decision.

If you doubt that hospitals actually misuse operational data in the ways just described, consider one more example. If you live in a large city, it is likely that some hospital in your area has announced its intention to drop out of the trauma network. A hospital spokesperson explains that the institution lost $5 million on the service during the prior year. This number, of course, is always based on fully allocated costs. To make the decision to leave the trauma network worthwhile, that hospital would have to lay off one hundred staff members (assuming $50,000 per staff member per year, including benefits)! It is unlikely, however, that the hospital will be able to lay off anything like one hundred FTEs, and chances are that it will be worse off after leaving the trauma network. There may be good reasons to withdraw, but this kind of thinking is not one of them.

The Shape of a New Management Paradigm

Just as there was a continuity of care imperative driving the new patient care organization, there is a continuity imperative in the executive suite of the future hospital. This is a potentially scary prospect for administrators, since the skills that will be needed for success tomorrow are not the same as for today. Not everyone who begins this journey will find a comfortable role within the new organizational structure.

This structure can be thought of as a two-way undertaking.

We must rethink what we want our senior managers to be accountable for. At the same time, we need to align authority and responsibility with that new notion of accountability. Simply put, we want most of our senior managers to be accountable for the care, quality, and financial performance of services provided to specific groups of patients and to be responsible for patients' satisfaction. It is not sufficient to redeploy and cross train our work force and assemble teams at the bedside, only to have them still negotiate with the complex matrix of our current departmental management structure. There must be a radical departure from a nearly total reliance on functional groupings and hierarchies as our overriding organizational principle.

Table 5.2 provides a glimpse of a new management structure that is derived from the principles of patient-focused care at the bedside, the need to rethink groupings of patients, and the imperative that in any rational management structure we must match authority and responsibility. The fundamental difference between this structure and our current model should be obvious: we have doubled the percentage of resources that we expect to manage directly at the bedside. The result is that the new patient care centers will not merely *coordinate* most nonnursing activities for their patients but they will also *own* and control 70 to 80 percent of all the services their patients routinely require. A surgical unit, for example, will provide both the nursing care that their

Table 5.2. Vision of Resource Allocation.

Administration (10%) Top Management and Administrative Activities	
Central Services (15%–20%) Services exhibiting demonstrable scale Expensive equipment or highly skilled personnel lacking critical mass in a single unit Facility-related services	*Operating Units* (70%–75%) Nursing care—all levels Operating and recovery rooms and personnel (if surgery) Routine ancillary procedures Patient support functions Patient-related clerical and administrative activities

patients need (as they do today) and routine ancillaries (basic lab and X ray), pharmacy, housekeeping, transportation, admitting, certain medical records functions, and so forth. These actions will not be organized by a matrix, but the staff will be run, hired, fired, and evaluated by unit management. An example can help us to discover why this must be so.

Let us say that you have been told that in the future your title will not be vice president—support services, but rather vice president of mommies and babies. In your new job, you will be held accountable for virtually everything involving maternity patients at the hospital: the services that they receive, their length of stay, their satisfaction, medical staff relationships, pricing parameters, overall clinical quality, staff turnover, and bottom-line results. This sounds like a good idea—a far cry from the seemingly random bundle of departments that you have been trying to manage for the past few years.

Then you spend a nearly sleepless night trying to figure out how you will do this new job. The answer soon occurs to you: they will have to give you the resources and the authority to do the job right, or you will not accept. You will not be held accountable for all those functions if you have to negotiate for everything your patients need using a hopeless maze of departments.

The next day, you lock yourself in your office and have your secretary cancel all meetings and hold all your calls. (Being vice president has its perks.) You start to make a list of activities that you will need to design and control to make the new job responsibilities manageable.

- Your customers will not wait for an hour or more on the first floor in a place called the admitting office for processing. Furthermore, you won't tolerate $200,000 per year in allocated costs to accomplish these tasks for your patients. You will "own" the admitting function for mommies and babies.

- You will not negotiate for thirty different people to be assigned randomly in the course of a year to get your customers' rooms cleaned and bed linens changed.
- Your patients will not be transported to a central department for ultrasound studies. Furthermore, these are needed often enough that even a centrally dispatched solution would be unresponsive to your doctors' needs. That routine service must be available on the unit.
- Because the daily "clocks" of your patients may depend on when they delivered, a rigid meal-time schedule dictated by the dietary department may not be adequate. You make a note to investigate alternatives.
- Medical records assembly and coding for your patients will be straightforward. You really only need a medical records department for archiving. Your nursing staff members will code their own charts during the slow periods that are inevitable in the maternity business.
- You see no reason to be at the scheduling mercies of a centralized IV team—nor do you want their costs allocated to your unit. Your nursing staff members will do this themselves.

This is the kind of thinking that occurs when we focus on groups of patients and match authority and responsibility. Eventually, the vice president of mommies and babies will also begin to work with the nursing staff to explore different models for staffing and care.

A Broader Application

The example just given may seem very selfish. It may appear to ignore the greater good of the hospital in deciding which costs may be allocated to a particular patient care center and which ones may not be. If all units acted like that, a few might be saddled with the bulk of the allocated costs from centralized departments. That would not be fair.

We need to understand that the new paradigm actually pushes this concept housewide. There will not be just a vice president of mommies and babies; we will make that role the template for the majority of our line management structure. We may therefore name vice presidents for surgery, ambulatory care, hearts–critical care, orthopedics-neurology, and so forth. Each of these senior executives will be authorized to evaluate every function needed by their patients in a "make-buy" framework. What follows from this process is the need to restructure what remains of the centralized departments and to refashion their roles in some cases. We can speculate about what might happen to certain centralized departments at the end of such a process.

Housekeeping (as a department) will be much smaller in most hospitals. Daily room cleaning is likely to be provided by multiskilled staff in each patient care center. Some other areas, like radiology and the operating rooms, may also decide to do their own routine cleaning. Housekeeping as we now know it may consist of a small crew of people, headed by an executive housekeeper. The crew would always be busy, waxing floors on a fixed monthly schedule and cleaning public and common areas on a daily basis. The executive housekeeper's role would become truly "executive" in nature; there would be very little time spent on direct supervision. The key responsibilities of the position would shift to defining what "clean" means at the hospital; recommending cleaning techniques, products, and frequencies; establishing training programs; and monitoring compliance with hospitalwide standards (in essence, making sure that the vice president of mommies and babies does not balance the budget of the unit at the expense of cleanliness or infection control).

We can also speculate about the kind of change that might occur in a large professional department, such as respiratory therapy. Since much of its high-volume, low-tech work would be absorbed into other positions within the patient care centers, it is likely that the professional therapists' lives would change. They would likely be deployed directly to the areas that consume the vast majority of their most sophisticated care: the critical care units of the hospital. There they might become full-time, permanent members of the care teams. There would also be a role for some of them in designing training programs for the cross-trained staff, perhaps delivering the curriculum and conducting quality reviews housewide.

We will deal with deployment decisions and job design more extensively in later chapters. These examples are presented to give some early insights into the management imperatives that result from the new paradigm.

What It Takes to Be A Successful Manager

For those of you who might have thought that patient-focused restructuring was going to involve a lot of redeployment and cross training of staff but leave the traditional management structure in place, the preceding sections must have come as quite a shock. The vice president of mommies and babies does not sound anything like the position you or any of your colleagues trained for. Moreover, it places a new and strong emphasis on hands-on management of day-to-day operations of a nearly full spectrum of functional areas. This is not the traditional set of skills that future CEOs necessarily concentrate on.

Many of us (including the author) were prepared by the M.B.A.-M.H.A. curriculum to become health care executives in the traditional mold. This process essentially prepared us to become "superintendents" or "deans," not hands-on managers of the departments that we were called upon to lead. The "dean" analogy is particularly appropriate (especially in large hospitals).

In the academic world, when one becomes a dean, the job entails directing the activities of a group of often varied experts. For example, if you are a dean of liberal arts, you will have a dizzying array of specialist departments reporting to you. Although your own expertise may be in English history, the departments of music, German, English literature, and social sciences are likely to be included in the college of liberal arts. As an English history expert, you will probably not get closely involved in the running of, say, the music department. Issues of curriculum design, teaching methods, or even the selection of faculty are likely to be left with the department itself. You will concern yourself with overall budgeting, facilities, and management of the size and balance of the tenured faculty.

Hospital management has more parallels to this system than we might like to admit. Consider a vice president of professional services (ancillary departments). The basic management approach today seems to be something like this: "I'm a lay manager. You're a director of pharmacy. I don't know much about pharmacy, so here's what we'll do. If my phone doesn't ring off the hook with complaints about service and your personnel costs don't increase by more than 6 percent a year, you look good, and I look good. Okay?" This implicit "deal" is cut with each department under the vice president's purview.

This example is clearly exaggerated to make a point, but there is a great deal of truth in it (although the smaller the hospital, the harder it is for management to operate this way). Other industries do not work this way. If you are a fresh young M.B.A. hired into a management training program by a large manufacturer, your first posting might be as an assistant plant manager at a company production facility. Your view of your role and your own development would almost certainly lead you to learn how each machine in the plant operates—its throughput, its set-up time, its maintenance requirements, things that can go wrong, and the way it fits into the total production process. In fact, you would probably be fired if you failed to acquire this knowledge (and perhaps operate some of the machinery) during your first six months on the job.

Think about hospital managers. With the rare exception of someone with a background in medical technology, it would be unheard of to imagine that the vice president of professional services might actually know how to operate the Coulter Counter in the hematology lab. Learning its costs, functionality, capabilities, set-up requirements, throughput, and self-diagnostic features might take a day or two, but the experience would demystify the process for you. It might even start you thinking about how its capabilities could be more widely distributed in the hospital. You might want to find out why you need a college degree and certification to operate the machine in some states. The analogy can also be applied to the laundry, medical records, EKG, and the whole armamentarium of hospital services.

The new model needs managers with such skills and sensibilities. Yes, managing health care services is different from overseeing a manufacturing operation. But we should not let the science and mystery overwhelm us. The vast majority of the issues at play (and that are important for management) are accessible to anyone with reasonable intelligence, an open mind, and common sense. We should observe, ask questions, and listen, as well as evaluate critically the received wisdom that is often placed in the path of understanding and change.

The new paradigm represents fundamental change in the magnitude of the hospital's resources, their allocation, and management. It will demand different skills from our work force and our managers and executives. The benefits of this admittedly scary magnitude of change are commensurate with the risks and include better care and service for patients, lower costs, and an enhanced sense of ownership and involvement for our employees. Now that we have laid the foundation for the restructuring initiative, the next three chapters will begin to deal with "how-to" issues entailed in designing and implementing the operational components of the new order.

6

Patient Aggregation: From Nursing Units to Patient Care Centers

This chapter addresses the question of how we decide which businesses to manage in the patient-focused hospital. At this point, we know several important features of the patient-focused paradigm as they relate to the grouping of patients, desired services at the bedside, management arrangements, and even bed size and critical mass. The next level of detail we need in order to make specific deployment decisions and design new processes and jobs involves the analysis of patient types and specific service demands to create coherent aggregations of patients for whom we can customize appropriate operating environments.

Before launching into this area in detail, we should remind ourselves of one very important imperative of the new system. Operating leverage—the means of improving performance—for ourselves and our customers results from capitalizing on differences, not from the forced engineering of similarities. Put another way: in creating new aggregations of patients, we are not attempting to find a better one-size-fits-all operating approach; we are seeking, where possible, different sets of patient needs around which we can design distinct operations. As you will see, we will likely arrive at four or five different operational models for hospitals of two hundred beds or more. For smaller hospitals, there will probably be fewer; in very small hospitals, perhaps only one.

Two additional introductory observations are required. First, any specific examples or illustrations used here or in subsequent chapters are not the "right" answers. They are simply what the demands at specific hospitals have pointed to as local solutions. The principles and tools, not the particular outcomes, are the important dimensions of the discussion in this chapter. Second, most of the patient-focused work to date has centered on inpatients. Consequently, the bulk of this chapter is devoted to this portion of hospital activities. There is now enough early design experience, however, to allow some speculation on outpatient demand models and their implications for the growing ambulatory care side of the business.

Where To Begin?

There are many ways to look at the service needs of our patients. Most hospitals today decide that the best means of addressing patient care requirements is to group patients by their medical need: orthopedics, obstetrics, urology, cardiology, cardiac surgery, and so forth. This approach is reckoned to be both appropriate and expedient; it allows the clustering of specific physicians' patients and experienced nursing resources. Even in the new system, this will turn out to be a useful guideline in many situations. But it has limitations, as the following two examples illustrate.

Many larger hospitals establish oncology units for inpatients. On the surface, this practice is quite sensible. Diagnostically similar patients are clustered for internal operating effectiveness, and, perhaps more importantly, a marketable entity is created (a cancer center). But the diagnostic similarity of the patients may not actually generate any operating leverage for the hospital. In terms of clinical and other patient needs, cancer can mean many things. Consider first the variety of patients who might be accommodated on an oncology unit (assuming that all cancer patients are admitted to that unit today).

- Patients who feel fine but have, say, a chronic, mild cough and are admitted for a biopsy.
- Patients who are sent home after a biopsy, with a more or less clean bill of health.
- Patients whose biopsy was followed by a radical neck procedure. After surgery, these patients' needs may have more in common with a trauma case than a generic oncology case. Their needs are driven by their postoperative care requirements. The fact that the surgery was due to cancer may have little to do with their immediate (physical) care.
- Patients needing relatively straightforward surgery who will be discharged in good condition within two or three days.
- Patients in for an overnight stay involving chemotherapy and the management of possible side effects.
- Patients in the terminal stages of their disease, receiving anything from around-the-clock critical care to hospice-like services.

In essence, oncology presents in microcosm the entire range of hospital services—medical, surgical, low intensity, high intensity, and even critical care (both medical and surgical). The problem is compounded if we take a more longitudinal view of the course of cancer. For many patients, cancer is a five-year (or more) experience. We tend to think of the inpatient side more than other dimensions. For the patient, however, cancer is likely to be viewed as five years of outpatient needs, punctuated by several inpatient episodes. The ambulatory component is a nearly endless series of visits for initial workups and diagnosis, chemotherapy, radiation therapy, follow-up exams, and episodes of "worry" (understandably, almost any ache or pain is likely to result in an office visit and diagnostic work to rule out further spread of the disease). There may be good reasons for establishing cancer centers, but operating leverage is not likely to be one of them.

The other side of this argument is illustrated by similarities between apparently dissimilar patients. Just as some clinical categorizations may mask profound differences, some traditionally distinct types of patients may in fact present opportunities for operating leverage and tailored services. Consider two types of patients: long-term medical patients and total hip replacement patients (orthopedics). What many of these patients have in common is that they are bedridden. This fact alone can be the primary determinant of the amount of work these patients represent for hospital care givers. The fact that they must have their beds changed while still in them, receive bed baths, and use the bed pan are likely to affect nursing's work load much more than, say, how many IV bags are attached to their arms or how many dressing changes they require. This perspective also has implications for the type of staff and the skill mix that we would need to care for these patients.

Therefore, though we should begin our aggregation analysis with traditional clinical designations, we should not stop there. The opportunities that we will miss and the complexities involved suggest a more micro-level approach.

Diagnosis-Related Groups and Medical Diagnostic Categories

Two other categorizations of patients are also in common use today—diagnosis-related groups (DRGs) and medical diagnostic categories (MDCs). These are both useful ways of organizing data, but each presents major shortcomings as the sole or primary determinant of patient aggregations under a model of patient-focused care.

There are 490 DRGs used to classify patients today. They have their origins in the financial realm. Originally developed by the State of New Jersey, DRGs were adopted by Medicare as a means of determining prospectively the amount of money a hospital would be paid for treating a particular patient. In some states and localities, Blue Cross, Medicaid, and even commercial payers have adopted or adapted this methodology. As with most things in life, the eighty-twenty rule generally applies. Roughly 80 percent of hospital patients are represented by about 20 percent of all possible DRGs, but that figure still represents nearly one hundred different possibilities. Furthermore, there can still be considerable variation within a specific DRG, especially when applied to both Medicare and younger patients (a seventy-year-old patient having his gallbladder removed can be quite different from a thirty-five-year-old having the same procedure, even when both procedures are deemed uncomplicated).

MDCs, of which there are twenty-three, are much broader categories. MDCs essentially deal with body systems (for example, musculo-skeletal) and disease processes. All DRGs can be mapped into MDCs. Whereas the problem with DRGs was their total number (in spite of which they can still ignore important differences), the difficulty posed by MDCs is that they are too general in nature and, more importantly, subsume vast differences in patient care needs. The oncology example used earlier is an apt analogy for the way that MDCs typically aggregate patients. Under the heart and circulatory MDC, for example, we will find patient conditions ranging from arrhythmia and high blood pressure to angioplasty and even open-heart surgery.

Although both DRGs and MDCs have deficiencies as an existing and handy way to aggregate patients in the new paradigm, they are in a sense on the right track. We need something that approaches the simplicity of MDCs but also provides a means for distinguishing among patients more finely—a methodology that takes into account similarities of resources and care processes.

Patient Types—A Useful Middle Ground

Patient types is a none-too-snappy term for a methodology that converts the maze of 490 DRGs into forty-six categories of patients. The model is based on the understanding that we need to seek similarities in patients beyond the traditional clinical service designations generally used to define nursing units. As we have seen, these designations can be simultaneously too narrow and too broad: too narrow in the sense that they can overlook similarities of care processes and resources (for instance, separating general surgery and urology) and too broad in the sense that they aggregate potentially very different patients (for example, grouping both disc repairs and head trauma as neurosurgery). Combined with the shortcomings of both DRGs and MDCs, this situation required a new system for categorizing patients that would present hospital management with better, understandable data.

Let us review in some detail the dimensions that can allow us to judge similarities among patients (in addition to the traditional and still important dimension of nursing expertise). *"Schedulability"* and *predictability* are measures of our ability to anticipate the arrival and the needs of a patient. In general, patients who are both schedulable and predictable are our easiest customers to satisfy—*if* we develop a tailored operating approach focused on their needs. Most elective surgery cases and even some medicine cases (overnight chemotherapy patients, for example) fall into this group. Few patients are schedulable but unpredictable, but quite a few patient types are unschedulable and predictable (for example, normal deliveries).

Length of stay encompasses several factors, not the least of which is our ability to provide continuity of care throughout a patient's stay. In general, the shorter the stay, the better we are able to design operating approaches that deliver high levels of continuity with care givers. The longer the stay, the more difficult this objective becomes (because of the traditional five-day work week). Also, as length of stay increases, it is possible that some patients may move into a different category—the beginning of their stay being, say, surgical in nature and the latter portion more medical or rehabilitative. Taken together, schedulability-predictability and length of stay can be powerful determinants of patient aggregations. Though no hospital has yet made this part of its patient-focused restructuring, one could imagine a patient care center where the primary criterion for admission would be a 95 percent probability that the patient will be discharged by

Friday at 3:00 P.M. Such a unit could then be closed for six shifts (until Monday mornings). The savings could be immediate and substantial.

Deficits in patients' *activities of daily living*, as mentioned earlier, can be the most significant determinant of "work" for some patients. This dimension also has significant implications for skill mix, especially for bedridden (but not necessarily critically ill) patients. Patterns of *ancillary service consumption* need to be considered since deploying lab and X ray services to the patient care centers should be capable of meeting 80 percent or so of the clustered patients' needs. Ancillary services in this context include physical therapy. *Physician convenience* is also an important aggregation criterion. We do not want the doctors having to travel to more units in the future than they do today to attend to their patients. In reality, this turns out to be a fairly easy goal to meet, since in most larger hospitals doctors' patients are not nearly as neatly distributed or concentrated as our unit designations might lead us to believe.

These factors, as well as the direct nursing care involved with particular patients, have been used to develop profiles of care for each kind of patient's stay. Figure 6.1 shows several examples of the care flow and resource consumption patterns using this framework. All of the profiles were then analyzed to develop reasonably coherent patient types, listed in Table 6.1. Clearly, most of the patient types coincide with common sense notions of patient similarities and do not appear to present any radical new categorizations. This is a useful outcome because we will not usually have to debate the reasonableness of the model.

Creating the Building Blocks

Before we can begin to look at possibilities for patient care centers, we need to add some hard numbers to the analysis. We must discover how many patients of each type are in the hospital at any given time. This involves mapping average daily census by DRG into the patient types. Figure 6.2 shows the results of this

Table 6.1. Patient Types.

Major general surgery
Minor general surgery
ENT surgery
Open-heart surgery
Angina/chest pain
Myocardial infarction
Other cardiology
Cardiac catheterization
Thoracic surgery
Vascular surgery
Vascular medical
Transient ischemic attack
Other neurology
Neurosurgery
Major ortho surgery
Minor ortho surgery
Fractures
Other ortho medical
General medical
GI medicine
ENT medical
AIDS/Infectious disease
Diabetes
Burns
Pneumonia and bronchitis
Chronic obstructive pulmonary disease
Other pulmonary medical
Oncology medical
Oncology surgical
Chemotherapy
Radiation therapy
GYN surgery
GYN medical
Vaginal delivery
Caesarean delivery
Antepartum complications
Normal newborn
Neonatal
Pediatric surgical
Pediatric medical
Mental disorders
Substance abuse
Orthopedic rehab
Neurology rehab
Hospice
Infection/Inflammation

Figure 6.1. Patient-Type Profiles.

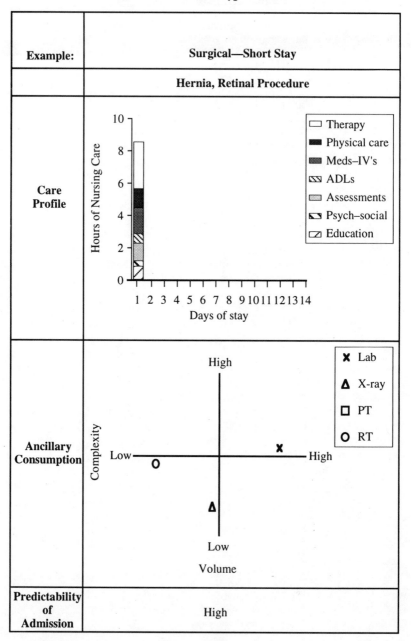

Figure 6.1. Patient-Type Profiles. Cont'd.

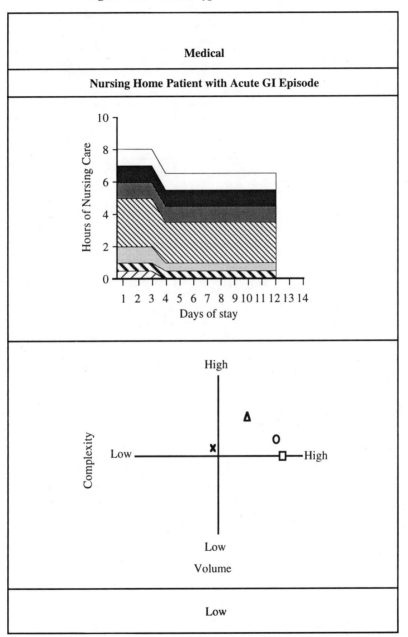

Figure 6.2. Distribution of Patient Types.

Specialty	Average Census	Inpatient Types		
Cardiology	25	Open-heart surgery 14	Myocardial infarction 4	Other cardiology 3
Medicine	30	General medicine 7	Pneumonia 5	Gastro-intestinal 4
		Pulmonary 2	Ear–Nose–Throat 1	Diabetes 1
OB/GYN	27	Normal delivery 12	Gynecological surgery 8	C-section 5
Orthopedics	15	Surgery (major) 10	Surgery (minor) 3	Fractures 1
Surgery	44	General (major) 21	General (minor) 12	Ear–Nose–Throat 5
Newborn	29	Neonate 18	Normal newborn 11	
Pediatrics	8	Medicine 6	Surgery 2	
Other	40	Rehabilitation 16	Psychiatry 18	Substance abuse 6
Total	**218**			

Figure 6.2. Distribution of Patient Types. Cont'd.

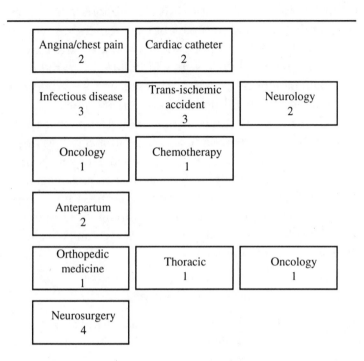

analysis for a 300-bed hospital. Note that not all forty-six patient types are represented and that several categories are quite small. This will almost always be the case. It is also important to realize that in aggregating demand into patient care centers we will be concerned with the 80 percent of patients who are fairly easy to group together. The smaller clusters will be fitted into the margins of the main patient care centers. This practice is no different than current attempts to "fill up" various nursing units.

As with many of the tools in this book, the patient types outlined here should be seen merely as one rational way to organize the data needed to make decisions. Smaller hospitals may not need to resort to this methodology, and larger hospitals may wish to develop their own. Moreover, renaming DRGs and grouping them into patient types accomplishes nothing more than organizing patient demand into categories that we can work with in defining patient care centers.

Confronting Reality

It may already have been obvious that this discussion about reaggregating patients and defining new and coherent patient care centers would eventually be forced to take into account the constraints created by the existing hospital facility. These can be wide ranging.

- The hospital is laid out with only fifteen to twenty-five beds per floor.
- The hospital has fifty beds per floor, but no seemingly related grouping of patient types adds up to even thirty patients.
- The hospital has a total of only sixty beds.
- Some logical groupings are obvious, but several of them exceed the capacity of any floor.
- Your physicians have historically insisted on locating certain patients together (for example, oncology of all sorts), even though you now know there is little or no operating leverage available through their aggregation.

There is no single solution to these problems. The work of defining new patient care centers is probably equal measures of art and science within the constraints of a given structure. Beyond some renovations, most hospitals cannot realistically consider reconfiguring their bed floors as part of the initial wave of patient-focused restructuring. However, there are some guidelines and suggestions for what is possible within the commonly found constraints.

Geography and layout are not usually major obstacles. It is possible to manage one patient care center on two adjacent floors. This is being done today on a thirty-bed orthopedics unit at a major academic medical center. This unit consists of two fifteen-bed floors of a round building—far from ideal but workable through good management.

Not all of the patients on a given center need to be of the same type, although their needs should be related as much as possible. On a forty-bed surgical patient care center, it is possible to have several "clusters" only interrelated by some of their bedside activities. Such units do not require nurses to be generalists across the entire spectrum of the unit. In fact, in most cases, the majority of the care givers work with a fairly narrow range of patient types. However, a handful of staff members on such a mixed unit may be paid significantly more for having extremely broad skills and the ability to "plug in" to a range of teams when the work load varies. One hospital refers to this highly skilled staff as the SWAT team.

In small hospitals, there may be only one patient care center. If the hospital has only one story, this approach actually has advantages since ancillary redeployment is not really an issue. Within such a patient care center, clinical clusters (as just described) will probably be used but under a one-unit management regime.

Not all decisions about patient care centers will be as tidy as we might like. There are going to be areas requiring trade-offs between internal operating leverage and external factors. For instance, in the case of oncology, a hospital might choose one of two available options: (1) an inpatient-based cancer center that might sacrifice operating leverage for market impact or (2) an outpatient-based center that also tracks inpatients who might be distributed across many units in the hospital.

Defining patient care centers is probably the most technically difficult task for many hospitals in their restructuring efforts. The answers and options will not be obvious (especially at the margin), and political barriers and physical constraints will always result in some suboptimization. The good news is that experience shows that a wide variety of configurations can render major benefits, even where they fall short of some theoretical ideal.

A Real Example

Although as of this writing no hospital has fully implemented the concept of patient-focused care for all inpatients, many have developed long-term visions of the way they will aggregate and manage their patients and the resources required for their patients' care. This section examines the factors involved at one particular hospital in its development of a long-term deployment and aggregation plan for inpatient services.

The hospital in question operates about seven hundred beds and offers the full range of acute-care services that would be expected in a regional medical center of that size—including open-heart surgery. The design of the hospital is more "horizontal" than most, that is, patient floors are large, and each is capable of accommodating about 120 patients (in three forty-bed units). Administrators' analysis of their patients' needs resulted in the creation (on paper) of five patient care centers, each with fairly distinct patient requirements and clear implications for different operating approaches. Some of the decisions necessarily involved compromises, and some decisions were deferred until the experience of implementing the first unit or two could provide feedback.

The five patient care centers (essentially, minihospitals) that this institution developed as its long-term plan are the following:

1. General surgery and specialty services
2. Orthopedic and neurological care
3. Cardiovascular center
4. Family care services
5. Oncology and diagnostic medicine

Their sizes range from 100 to 130 beds, and each center is to occupy a different floor. The proposal includes management realignment as well, such that each floor-center would ultimately be under the control of a single executive.

On the surface, the organization of these centers does not seem to violate any of our usual ideas about how inpatients ought to be grouped in a modern hospital—partly because their sizes mask some new ideas and because their names do not communicate adequately what is to be included on each floor or the operating approach implied for them. Furthermore, since this hospital neither serves a large indigent population nor has a large trauma service, some of the demand-aggregation challenges we might expect at a hospital of its size are not present. Nevertheless, this vision does provide a fairly clear example of the issues at work in defining patient care centers. Let us look briefly at each of these minihospitals.

General and special surgery. This is where the vast majority of all short-stay surgery patients will be cared for. The operating approach will focus on the schedulability of admissions, maximum continuity of care, predictable postoperative care requirements, minimum documentation, and rapid recovery for discharge. Ancillary service requirements are routine and fairly concentrated. Most operating room resources would report to this center. The staffing model has to be fairly flexible to allow for the usual decline in census over the weekend.

Orthopedics and neurology. This center will accommodate longer-stay patients with significant deficits in the activities of daily living (ADL) and with rehabilitation requirements. Partly because of the longer stays, bedside care will be less intense than on the surgery unit; because of the ADL deficits, the skill mix may be somewhat less rich. Streamlined documentation will be possible for most patients. And because about 80 percent of demand at this hospital originates with these patients, physical therapy (PT) and occupational therapy (OT) will report through this center's management structure and eventually locate most of their resources on the unit. PT and OT will still provide care to patients elsewhere, but their main focus will be here. Other ancillary services will be nominal, with the probable inclusion of EEG. (The exclusion of neurosurgery from this unit is intentional. At this hospital, most neurosurgery is elective and/or spine and is included in the surgery patient care center).

Hearts and critical care. This center will accommodate almost all of the hospital's critically ill patients and those requiring intensive care (medical and surgical). Heart patients represent a large percentage of this population. Eventually, a large proportion of the beds on this floor will be capable of intensive and critical care, a situation that will minimize the need to transfer patients between different levels of care. These transfers today create high cost (multiple pockets of fixed costs) and compromised continuity of care. The bulk of the hospital's professional respiratory care resources will be integrated into this patient care center. Charting and data base management will likely be automated, as will the complex protocols of care for these patients. The skill mix will be rich. Ancillaries will be only slightly different than today; we already tend to bring services to these patients rather than transporting them to the central departments.

Family care services. This floor houses most of the hospital's low-intensity services and includes maternity, pediatrics, and psychiatry. This center is clearly not as coherent as the others, although it is not as bad as it sounds. Essentially, the floor will include three discrete care environments, sharing resources wherever possible. The good news is that maternity and psychiatry are already fairly self-contained and reasonably independent of the rest of the hospital (no huge requirements for lab, X ray, or operating rooms, for instance). Sharing of nursing resources will be minimal.

Medical diagnostic services and oncology. This is the center for the majority of medical patients, including medical oncology (surgical oncology is distributed according to the type of surgery). Here the population is generally older, with complicating conditions and disabilities being common. The clinical challenge is significant, compounded by ADL deficits. Ancillary needs are complex early in patient stays, but it is generally not economical to redeploy MRIs, CATs, and gamma cameras. Opportunities to streamline documentation will be harder to implement than in procedure-intensive centers.

A few observations are needed to conclude this example. First, not all patient care centers will present the same opportunities for operating leverage. In this example, most of the leverage is in the first three units; the family care center and medical center are less rich in possibilities. This limitation is perfectly acceptable and likely to be the case in most hospitals. Second, to maintain continuity of care and minimize the need to transfer patients between centers, monitoring capabilities will probably be available on all appropriate units. For example, in one hospital 80 percent of the general surgery patients in intensive care units or step-down–type beds were there solely because of the need for monitoring (due to a history of or risk factors for cardiac complications), not because of their postsurgical condition. This capability could easily be distributed. In the long run, critical care capabilities may even be decentralized or at least available for patients on each center.

A Special Hybrid for Selected Patients

One group of patients is particularly difficult to cater to at the bedside: complex medical diagnostic patients. As we saw earlier in our discussion of demand characteristics, these patients consume a disproportionate percentage of high-cost ancillaries (MRI, CAT, special studies, and nuclear medicine). To meet their needs in a patient-focused way, we would like to put these capabilities closer to the bedside. However, the high cost of such machines, the space they require, and even their special shielding all conspire to make this redeployment extremely unlikely. Furthermore, outpatients provide the other major segment of demand for these services.

One hospital is contemplating something truly innovative for these patients as part of its long-range facility plan. It is investigating the feasibility of configuring a ten- to fifteen-bed "medical intake unit" located adjacent to the radiology department on the first floor of the hospital. Medical patients with significant diagnostic requirements would be admitted to this unit and stay for a day or two before being transferred to a more typical medical unit or discharged. This system sacrifices a bit of continuity of care but probably makes a good trade-off for the patients. It is during the first two days of stay that they are most likely to be "sick" and simultaneously subjected to a rigorous series of diagnostic procedures (mostly radiology-related). By locating these patients next to radiology, we can minimize their travel and waiting times. Furthermore, we accomplish this goal without duplicating expensive technology; outpatients could use the same facilities but gain access to them through different doors.

We are likely to see more creative ideas explored over the next few years. As the patient-focused paradigm spreads across the industry, we will see it evolve in new and exciting ways unanticipated by the pioneers. But this is part of the natural maturing of new ideas and the joy of participating in their evolution and growth. There will be no shortage of problems that need to be solved, even within the new order.

How Do Outpatients Fit In?

Most of the patient-focused restructuring work to date has concentrated on operating strategies for inpatients. Any new paradigm that cannot solve the inpatient cost and service problem will never gain any real traction in the industry, so it is reasonable to start with the traditional inpatient business (and its lion's share of the costs). But all the recent trends in hospitals point to a growing ambulatory care business—especially with continued advancements in surgical techniques and laser technology. For virtually every hospital in the country, outpatient revenue will represent an ever-increasing portion of the total enterprise. How do the concepts of patient-focused care apply to outpatient services?

The answer to that question is only now being explored by a handful of institutions, but some of the early insights are interesting enough to share in this context. The first chapter of this book presented two True-Life Adventures that focused on outpatient services. Actually, only the first story was true. The second was a speculation about what is possible. The cross-trained radiology technician who can also register patients, take payments, draw lab specimens, and perform EKGs is perfectly legal in every state. The model is also not without precedent since all of these duties are performed in countless doctors' offices every day by cross-trained staff members (sometimes with lesser qualifications than a radiology technician).

It would be a mistake, however, to use the second story as a model for implementation. It is on the right track, and many hospitals might indeed benefit from its suggestions. But we should not get caught up in the specifics. Let us review a list of patient-focused issues surrounding outpatient services.

- Outpatient areas usually suffer from the totally inappropriate extension of the one-size-fits-all approach of the hospital. Worse yet, this means an *inpatient* one-size-fits-all approach is applied to outpatients. For example, it is the rare outpatient procedure indeed that requires less time for its paperwork than for its actual performance. Look at how little different the outpatient admitting form of your hospital is from the inpatient form.
- Just as the inpatient operating structure is generally designed for the perceived effectiveness of hospital departments, outpatient care began with that viewpoint—and worse. Most outpatient operating approaches have been designed by seeking

answers to such questions as "How can we most easily perform all these outpatient X rays in our X ray department without disrupting our focus on inpatients?" In general, we have
not asked the right question: "What's the best way to meet
the needs of the outpatient customer segments?" Furthermore, we have sought to fit everything into a five-day-a-week,
nine-to-five kind of operation, ignoring the fact that inpatients
are "available" at least sixteen hours a day and many outpatients might prefer evening and weekend hours.

- Just as we saw that there was not *one* inpatient business, there
  is not just one outpatient business. We must think about the
  needs that patients present and the business systems we need
  to cater to the various segments of demand. An ambulatory
  surgery patient is very different from someone referred for
  a routine chest X ray—both in resources consumed and in
  clinical risks involved.

- For many patients, we may need to rethink our attitudes. Many
  outpatients are not "sick." They may be worried; they may
  be pressed for time; or they may be concerned about paying
  the bill. Our challenge for these kinds of patients is not the
  pure clinical dimension of their needs; it is more likely to
  revolve around service levels, costs, and speed.

Again, although the answers for outpatients are not completely clear at this point in the development of our paradigm,
there are two related and increasingly useful segmentation scenarios that appear to hold promise. One scenario uses services
as its major criterion and the other uses patient condition for
segmenting demand. The spectrum of outpatient services is then
treated as follows under the two scenarios.

The services segmentation looks at the nature of the procedures involved in each outpatient encounter. Under this scenario,
we get the following "businesses":

- *Quick diagnostics* involves individual or small bundles of routine services. These services are typically easy, low risk, high
  volume, of moderate cost, and provided on an unscheduled
  basis.

- *Scheduled diagnostics* involves usually just one procedure that is high cost (for example, MRI) and requires a scarce resource (the machine, for instance), thus leading to the need to schedule the work.
- *Ambulatory surgery* requires both the scheduling of the procedure and the precise orchestration of multiple resources.
- A *quick visit* involves a brief, low-level encounter with a physician. This may be all that is involved, or it may generate a quick diagnostic encounter as a follow-up. Between 60 and 80 percent of patients who pass through an average emergency room fall into this category.
- *Emergencies* are the urgent or emergent subset of today's emergency department demand; they comprise typically 20 to 40 percent of total visits.

Each of these segments can be thought of as offering clues about how we should tailor our operating approach—whether to schedule, how much paperwork is appropriate, which hours of operation are appropriate, and so forth. The second segmentation scenario seeks to be even more general in nature and looks at pre- and postvisit conditions of patients.

- *Patients feel essentially the same when leaving as when they arrived.* These are not risky encounters for us or major events in the lives of our customers. We draw some blood, take an X ray, or the like. For this segment of the patient population, the process should be as easy, quick, and seamless as possible.
- *Patients feel worse when they leave than when they arrived.* This category includes the ambulatory surgery business and other invasive procedures. We take a more or less healthy person and, while improving his or her overall clinical status, inflict discomfort and temporary dysfunction. Many of these patients have significant postprocedure care and resource requirements.
- *Patients feel better when they leave than when they arrived.* This is much of the quick-visit business. A patient comes in hobbling and leaves with a wrapped ankle, crutches, and a

prescription for a pain killer. The patients' needs are fairly uncomplicated; they consume few resources and entail little risk or complexity.

- *Patients do not leave, and they are either much better or dead.* This is an admittedly very crude way to describe the true emergency room business. It is also accurate. In general, true emergency patients are either admitted or die. They are at high risk, consume massive amounts of resources, and are utterly unschedulable.

Although these are entertaining intellectual exercises, their real value is in pointing the way toward new ways of doing business and capitalizing on the potential leverage to be gained from focusing on specific patient needs. In the True-Life Adventure in the first chapter, we saw one way to respond to the quick-visit, feel-the-same group: minimum paperwork, maximum continuity, fastest service, special hours of operation and so forth. We can also imagine a new way of working with these patients. Of the 60 to 80 percent of emergency department patients whose needs are not even urgent, a large percentage are likely to be represented by just a handful of common complaints. Problems such as sore throats (with and without fever), injured joints, contusions, flu-like symptoms, and the like may comprise one-half or more of the nonurgent segment. Today many hospitals recognize this fact and have instituted triage and fast-track care for such patients. They probably have not pushed the principle far enough, though. Even under most fast-track systems, patients encounter a triage nurse, a receptionist, a nurse who takes vital signs and a brief history, perhaps a transporter, an X ray technician, a phlebotomist, and a physician.

It may be possible to develop nursing-directed protocols of care for the most common complaints. If you twist your ankle at the local softball game, your encounter at the hospital might go like this. You would be greeted by a nurse who would do a brief assessment. Deducing your complaint to be minor and with few risks, the nurse would "admit you" using a short form; take your vital signs; examine your ankle; order your X ray, perhaps perform it (in some states and settings) and mount it on the light box; draft prescriptions for an anti-inflammatory and a pain killer; summon the physician to check the X ray and sign the prescriptions; wrap the ankle; counsel the patient on postdischarge care; and sign the patient out. Although this process may be nurse-intensive, it provides great continuity for the patients, conserves the time of physicians for patients needing their services, and reduces the need in the emergency department for many positions with high levels of structural idle time: clerks, transporters, X ray technicians, phlebotomists, lab technicians, and the like.

In the months and years ahead, we will learn much more about patient-focused care in the ambulatory setting. The area is ripe for innovation and will need to be included in any long-term restructuring plan. These tantalizing glimpses of the potential for improved customer service should serve as encouragement for any pioneering hospitals that wish to tackle these problems head on.

One of the revolutions inherent in patient-focused care is its view of how and what we should manage in our hospitals. Since we are not department stores or fast-food outlets, we do not usually have the luxury of deciding *what* we will do or "sell." But that fact does not mean that we cannot make important decisions about how to do the work and how to assure that it is well managed for our customers. Patient aggregation is one of the cornerstones of the new model—where we express our beliefs about patient care and customer service by the way we group patients to meet their needs in the best way we can. Because of the wide variety of patient types and needs, these decisions will always involve some art and some trade-offs—in addition to the science we can bring to the process. This area can be expected to produce some startling innovations and new insights in the years ahead, as we all gain more experience with the new model and its potential.

7

Initial

Deployment

Decisions

Paradigms, ideas, and insights are all well and good, but eventually we are going to have to *do* something. Implementation has many components and options, and these will be the subjects of the next two chapters. At this point, we have a good sense of the problems with the current operating approach and a solid foundation for the new patient-focused paradigm and the way it is going to affect the dimension of patient aggregation. This understanding provides the motivation for restructuring and the first broad strokes of a vision of what living in a different world will be like.

Moving forward with implementation requires a set of "enablers" and decision-making tools common to nearly all institutions and a process for mobilizing people to make patient-focused care a reality. This chapter deals with tools and experiences needed to chart the next level of detail in the restructuring effort—deployment models for the major functions of hospitals. Having used overall demand patterns to postulate future patient care centers, the next step in the process involves an overarching approach for making decisions about what services and functions will be redeployed to the centers. There is now enough experience in various settings to permit this chapter to contain nearly equal measures of theory and real-world examples.

Lessons in Ancillary Redeployment

Putting routine services closer to the bedside can seem a daunting task. Most of us have had some experiences with some aspect of this issue that do not exactly bode well for the success of a more aggressive initiative. We may recall the nightmare of bureaucracy involved in redeploying a simple lab procedure—such as simple glucose tests—to the nursing units. It probably entailed six months of meetings involving scores of staff members and produced not only ill will and mistrust but also a thick procedure manual. This outcome is discouraging, especially since we are now suggesting the redeployment of "real" laboratory work—not just something simple like glucose tests, which patients will do for themselves after they are discharged.

A useful first step in visualizing the process therefore is to separate what will be difficult from what will not. Some ancillary activities are completely foreign to bedside care givers; others involve restrictive regulations and laws. A brief experiential review of where our efforts will be rewarded and where we are likely to spend political capital without any commensurate return follows.

Phlebotomy and basic specimen prep should not be a big problem to redeploy—at least from a technical point of view. Nursing personnel at most hospitals already do this on offshifts and for stat work. Resistance usually comes in two forms. The nurses will say that they do not have the time to do it and the lab staff may say the nurses will not do it right (especially the labeling). Nevertheless, a demand analysis is likely to show that the typical nurse will only have to draw a handful of samples per shift; besides, as we move to restructuring work, we will create time for nursing by reducing that devoted currently to such tasks as documentation. The objections of the lab can only be handled by experience, aided by the fact that the care givers will now be accountable directly for their phlebotomy work.

EKG should also be fairly straightforward. The training of EKG technicians is not extensive, regulation is minimal, and the procedure is relatively uncomplicated. The capital cost of the equipment is not significant. Furthermore, outside of the critical care areas (where most patients are monitored anyway), the average care giver will probably be called upon less than once a day to perform this procedure for an inpatient.

Providing basic respiratory care (spirometry, oximetry, IPPB, oxygen therapy, and the like) at the bedside should not be a problem but increasingly is. When this work first started, the usual response of respiratory therapy (RT) to redeploying very basic services was "Thank you!" These tasks were generally uninteresting and unrewarding; they were the source of most complaints from nurses and doctors about missed treatments, and at many hospitals the department was only succeeding in meeting 80 to 90 percent of demand. This gratefulness faded over time as those in RT realized that at the end of the restructuring process their department might disappear. The basic, high-volume procedures might be performed by cross-trained staff at the bedside, and the vast majority of the professional therapists would be redeployed to critical care areas. The technical arguments against redeploying basic RT work are not persuasive, and there is minimal state regulation to slow you down (although the RT guild is trying to change this as quickly as possible in many states). Even if this is a struggle at your hospital, it is one worth pressing.

Pharmacy has not been the focus of any cross-training initiatives. The only issue here is redeploying the pharmacists themselves to the patient care centers. Pharmacists are generally enthusiastic about this. The only dispute seems to focus on the scope of work for the redeployed pharmacists. As with today's satellite pharmacies and floor pharmacists, they may want to restrict the work to initial orders and use the central pharmacy to do refills and daily deliveries. There is no persuasive reason to separate these activities. Experience shows that one pharmacist can meet all the drug needs (initial orders, refills, IV, and delivery) of thirty to forty general care patients on a given shift without clerks, technicians, or a central dispensary. Several patient-focused hospitals are using computerized dispensing machines to cover the off-shifts and weekends. A central operation of some sort probably will be needed (for ordering and warehousing, high-tech admixtures, off-hour coverage, retail sales, and the like), but it is unlikely to play a major role in day-to-day dispensing.

The basic issue in physical therapy (PT) at most hospitals will be whether to redeploy the bulk of the resources to a discrete patient care center, as in the orthopedics-neurology example cited earlier. Only a small percentage of other patients receive PT services as a rule. After a consult (or using an established protocol), basic PT can be administered by properly trained bedside care staff. These services are typically ambulation, gait training, and chest percussion (sometimes performed by RTs as well). Cross training for these services is not likely to be a major hurdle, either technically or politically.

One thing should be kept in mind as a general rule in redeployment discussions: there are two separate decisions involved—*where* a given function is performed, and *who* performs it. The first decision is one of almost pure operating strategy and can be made independent of the second issue. The "where" decision can be made on its own merits based on patient needs. The "who" question will almost always have to take into account local regulation. However, state regulations may not always be as restrictive as they seem on first reading. Many state statutes (especially those dealing with RT and PT) have a neat little paragraph near the end with something like the following wording: "Nothing in this act shall be construed as preventing the reasonable performance of such activities by other qualified individuals." This qualification was probably inserted so that physicians could perform the functions involved, if they chose to. However, these

clauses have also created leeway for more than one hospital looking to use cross training as part of their restructuring.

Routine laboratory procedures and chest and extremity
films in radiology are the areas most likely to present challenges
in the form of regulation, capital cost, space, and training. These
areas are where much of the time in planning for ancillary redeployment will be spent by hospitals seeking to restructure. The
next two sections address the issues that commonly arise in these
important spheres.

Ancillary Redeployment: X ray

First, we should remind ourselves that patient-focused restructuring cannot be implemented using a set of monolithic rules.
Rather, a set of principles, ideas, and tools for making things
better for our customers is needed. As such, there are multiple
possibilities for the operating structure of any given hospital; furthermore, different approaches can be employed to tailor the
concept to different patient care centers within a particular institution. Even if this were not the case, the variety of state regulations
and other guidelines necessarily limit the possibilities open to
any given hospital. These factors appear no more clearly than in
the effort to make decisions about the provision and deployment
of routine radiology and laboratory services in the patient-focused
hospital.

Let us begin with radiology, reminding ourselves that chest
films generally account for 50 to 60 percent of all inpatient X
rays. Extremity films add about 10 percent to the total. By and
large, these are the procedures that we have the greatest interest
in making readily available to patients, both to save cost and busy-
work and, more importantly, to save wear and tear on our patients
and attending physicians. Yes, there may be special cases in very
large hospitals where we might consider redeploying fluoroscopy
as well for large medical units, but we should keep our attention
on the main issue: the performance of very routine radiological
procedures. There is enough experience in restructured hospitals

and in countless doctors' offices to state categorically that there are no objective barriers to training a variety of care givers to perform basic radiology exams. Despite this fact, most states have enacted regulations that limit our ability to proceed. Where this is not the case (in Tennessee, for example), care givers have been trained (by radiology) to perform the routine procedures their patients need. Experience shows that the retake rates for these exams are no higher than for the same exams performed elsewhere in the hospital by radiology technicians. Where regulation prevents cross-training, however, there are a number of potential strategies.

- Though far from an ideal solution (since it still relies on remote resources unaccountable to the patient care center), radiology services can be dispatched. This process can either involve on-site equipment or portables—much like stat service today. Responsiveness and flexibility remain problematic, however.

- Using a dispatched radiology technician and on-unit equipment, services can be scheduled in blocks on the patient care center. This approach is not perfect either, but it is thinkable.

- Cross-training is a two-way street. It does not just mean training nurses staff to perform other duties; it can mean training radiology technicians to perform a range of patient care duties. One innovative hospital recruited (internally) radiology technicians for a surgical patient care center. They were trained to be the equivalent of licensed nurses, capable of performing 70 percent or more of all patient care tasks at the bedside. They function as direct care givers for the bulk of their workday. On the occasions when a film is needed, their beepers go off; the signal indicates that a patient is already in the unit's X ray suite. The technician steps down the hall, checks the positioning, checks the settings, clicks the machine, checks the film for clarity, and then returns to the bedside care team.

All of these approaches are aimed at minimizing the structural idle time and, simultaneously, the waiting time involved in routine X rays. The suggestions all flow from the premise that very few patient care centers will have sufficient demand to justify a full-time radiology technician on two shifts each day. A typical surgery unit of forty beds, for example, might only need a dozen (or fewer) films per day (but spread across two shifts). It would be very expensive indeed to have an X ray technician waiting in an exam room for five or six chest films to be ordered on a given shift. The option of training technicians to perform other unit duties for most of the day is especially elegant in this regard. We still pay these employees like radiology technicians, not licensed vocational nurses (LVNs) and get quite a bargain. We get our patients' X rays done while still receiving a full day's effort from each staff member. It may be surprising to learn that though cross-training will not be embraced by all (or even most) radiation technicians, the ones who are doing it find the broader participation in patient care to be very rewarding and would not go back to the radiology assembly line if given the opportunity.

Ancillary Redeployment: Laboratory Services

The laboratory presents a somewhat different set of issues and options when considering redeployment. We should begin by stating the obvious: beyond the technical and scientific factors, the lab differs from the X ray department in that it requires the transport of samples, not patients, to get its work done. This is an important difference because of concern about inconveniencing patients in the performance of routine ancillary procedures. The major problems today are that an alarming number of patients are awakened before dawn each day to draw samples for their lab work and, even so, attending physicians often find themselves forced to play games with the lab system to get results when they need them. Both of these problems stem from the same source: a one-size-fits-all service strategy in the centralized laboratory.

The patient-focused goal we seek in decentralizing routine lab services is to improve the responsiveness and flexibility of the system. In the process, we also hope to reduce significantly the infrastructure costs of drawing, logging, processing, and reporting out lab work. Laboratory services are generally just as regulated by the states as X ray services (in many cases, more stringently than the federal government's recent Clinical Laboratory Improvement Amendments [CLIA] regulations require). Nevertheless, there are a number of options in meeting the need for a fairly predictable range of tests that comprise 70 percent or more of routine demand. The equipment and space needed are fairly modest, even when central lab technology is duplicated on the units. The cost runs about $200,000 to $300,000 per minilab and can be accommodated in about three hundred square feet. This cost will likely decrease over time as more appropriate technology is brought to bear. Early implementers of the patient-focused concepts chose not to fight any technology battles over what equipment would be used in the minilabs and therefore replicated the current equipment (to permit comparisons of results and techniques).

As decentralized labs take hold, smaller and more focused technology will be more readily available and more economically attractive. Even now, there are machines the size of a telephone handset that can perform six or more common tests in ninety seconds on a capillary-tubeful of blood (with impressive comparability to larger machines). There are two obstacles to their widespread adoption: first, they only make sense if used by bedside care givers, not centralized or roving laboratory technicians; second, today's approach leads us to focus on the high reagent costs of new technology compared to the central lab. Over time, it is likely that these costs will decrease sharply, and hospitals will also realize that the true, total costs of the current centralized processing of routine lab work are much higher than suspected and that reagent costs may not be a serious deterrent to the proliferation of innovative, portable technologies. In making many decisions involving new paradigms, we will have to extricate ourselves from the economic assumptions of the old world. When the structure changes, so do the economic possibilities.

With that background, let us explore some of the options emerging from the experiences of early implementers of patient-focused concepts.

The most common model (because of state regulations) is to create a unit-based minilab with a dedicated technologist on day shift. Offshift demand is either handled by the central lab or an internal "regional" lab, serving several floors. Provided that the patient care center is at least forty beds or so, the lab demand keeps the lab technician fairly busy, although the work load still tends to peak in the early morning. To fill in the structural idle time of the technician, several hospitals have assigned various types of deferrable work—running the center's supply and inventory system, for instance. On one restructured maternity unit, the laboratory technologist assists with feeding in the nursery as the work load permits.

One hospital (in a state where it is legal) has trained care givers to perform their own lab work on the unit. The lab selected the equipment, designed the training curriculum, and delivered the courses. Lab personnel maintain and calibrate the machines and perform periodic quality assurance activities.

Several other hospitals have equipped minilabs on the patient care centers and now use visiting technologists (usually for about four hours a day). Still other hospitals have upgraded their tube systems and perform the tests in the central lab as stats. This approach will probably work for a while, but as more and more beds are converted to this system the costs may rise (or at least will not ever go down).

Finally, despite state regulations prohibiting nonlab staff members from performing tests, one creative hospital built a minilab, and the laboratory trained the care givers to do the work. Each sample was split; half was sent to the central lab and half used to run the test on the floor. Only the central lab result was used in the record, but the hospital kept a detailed comparative log of the results; it hoped to use the results to seek a change in the law (or at least receive a waiver). After six months, no results differed beyond machine tolerances. Although the point was proven, the state did nothing. Sadly, this hospital has ceased to use its minilab (only temporarily, one hopes).

One of the interesting (and unexpected) outcomes of decentralization of routine lab service (and to a certain extent X ray) is that utilization of the services has declined. Some might have feared that the ready availability of these services would lead to higher consumption rates. However, because lead times and turnaround times have been drastically reduced, physicians tend to be more comfortable taking "rifle shots" (making sequential diagnoses). In centralized labs, with four- to six-hour turnaround times, "shotgun blasts" are the common mode; it is easier to order everything that might possibly be needed all at once, since follow-up work will likely take another four-hour cycle. With minilabs on the patient care centers, doctors can choose a narrower set of tests, get the results in minutes, and follow up if necessary.

The major barrier to unit-based minilabs (and the exploitation of new technology as well) will continue to be state regulation of laboratory staff in hospitals. Reversing the trends of the last thirty years will not be easy, especially since the laboratory guild is working to make the regulations even more restrictive. Unfortunately, in fact, the initiative for patient-focused care seems to be causing these efforts to intensify. We can only hope that as experience in selected hospitals demonstrates the efficacy of decentralization and cross training, we will see the pendulum begin to swing back toward the use of good judgment and common sense. In their effort to maintain their control over even the simplest and most automated of tests, laboratory technicians seem to resemble elevator operators who insist on pushing the buttons of an automatic elevator or union electricians who claim that only they are qualified to change light bulbs.

A General Deployment Framework

Because of their highly regulated nature, the ancillary services just discussed have been treated as a separate issue from the

Figure 7.1. Restructuring Decision Tree.

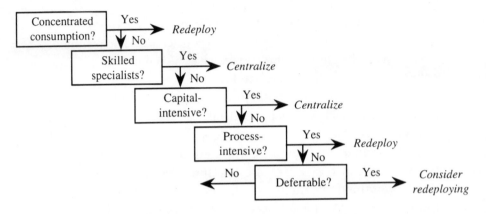

larger question of functional redeployment in the patient-focused hospital. Masked by the experiential discussion of those ancillary services, however, is the fact that the decisions involved are really part of a broader framework for evaluating the proper locations for all hospital functions. The analytical process for making deployment decisions is reasonably straightforward and involves a series of discrete questions and branches that make up the decision tree shown in Figure 7.1.

The five-step process does involve some complexity, judgment, calibration, and subtlety. It is not just something we can plug into a computer and then implement the results. Deployment in this context can be physical and managerial; we can redeploy a given function by physically moving it to one or more new locations and/or we can redeploy it by changing its position and set of relationships in the management structure. Also, what a function is needs to be defined rather narrowly in some contexts. For example, the hematology lab is not *a* function but rather a collection of interrelated activities, including, at a micro level, entry of orders, phlebotomy, accessioning, sample preparation, discrete tests (or groups of tests on a given machine), and the reporting of results, as well as all the other functions needed to provide and assure the accuracy of the service. Let us examine how the model works.

Step One. Is the Service Consumed by a Concentrated Patient Population?

This first question seeks to isolate the functions of the hospital that clearly need to be focused on specific groups of patients. For these activities, there is no reason to consider the other questions on the decision tree. Wherever possible, our new paradigm tells us, we want to locate services as close as possible to the patient. Some of the more obvious candidates for focused redeployment would include (at least in some hospitals)

- Physical and occupational therapy concentrated on orthopedics and neurology patients—if not physically (at first), then at least managerially. In some large medical centers, this approach might even result in a further segmentation, with portions of PT and occupational therapy focused on a sizable population of burn patients.
- The bulk of complex respiratory care services focused on critical care areas.
- The reporting relationships of the operating and recovery rooms restructured from a generic, functional reporting relationship to one associated with the majority of the hospital's surgical beds and resources.
- Specific people doing specific tasks. For example, an enterostomal therapist might be transferred organizationally out of the central nursing structure to the general surgery patient care center (where most of the stoma patients are likely to originate).
- A CAT scanner and MRI located on a new neurology-spine-orthopedics floor housing over one hundred patients (as will be tried at one large medical center).

Not surprisingly, not very many functions will fall into this special category since one of the legitimate reasons that hospitals centralized functions in the first place was to recognize that demand was broadly distributed; most patients got at least a little bit of nearly everything.

Step Two. Is the Function Performed by a Limited Number of Highly Skilled Specialists?

This is a tricky step. The key is to define what highly skilled means and to evaluate whether that level of skill is in fact appropriate. Otherwise we run the risk of keeping many activities centralized that could be appropriately redeployed. On the one hand, Coulter Counters are generally operated by highly skilled personnel; on the other hand, this amount of training may not be required by either local regulation or objective analysis. In most cases, the question is likely to boil down to an issue of total demand; a small number of highly skilled specialists often translates directly into modest demand levels for the service involved. We should also realize that this issue is not confined to clinical specialists; it could (and often does) apply to executives (for example, the CFO) and technicians and scientists (such as ethicists, biomedical engineers, or even plumbers and electricians).

For many hospitals, not too many major functions will be eliminated from consideration for redeployment at this point, particularly if care is taken to evaluate the necessity of the current level of skill of employees performing the task in question.

Step Three. Is the Function Capital Intensive?

Another tricky step. *Capital intensity* is, first of all, a relative term, not an absolute one. It is relative to the size of the institution, the volume of services delivered, and the opportunity for improvement in cost and/or service performance. Spending $250,000 on a new general radiology machine sounds capital-intensive. But if that expenditure eliminated even one position somewhere in the hospital (at, say, $30,000 per year, fully loaded), it would be cost-neutral, assuming a useful life of seven to ten years for the equipment. Furthermore, if it were used twenty-five times each day and had the potential to reduce length of stay by .25 day and improve patients' and doctors' perceptions of service levels, it could be quite a bargain indeed. The other complicating aspect of the term capital intensive is that it is often rooted in a particular time and technology. For example, redeploying large multichannel chemistry analyzers might present insurmountable capital barriers, but a newer, smaller, more focused technology might be perfectly feasible. The lesson to be learned here is that we must consider not only the current structure and technology but also emerging alternatives. In many hospitals, the list of patient-care activities that will be deemed capital intensive is likely to be rather small. Most functions will survive this question and remain in play for decentralization.

One other dimension of capital intensity needs to be mentioned: space. This is a particularly important consideration when looking at such items as laundry and dietary services. In addition to whatever investment we may have made in particular equipment and machinery, also involved is considerable (and difficult to reuse) square footage, often with special configurations (such as ceiling heights, external access, and adjacencies) and utilities (such as gas, high voltage, water, and ventilation). Eventually, hospitals may wish to examine the possibility of decentralizing these two services (especially dietary), but such options are likely to be deferred for some time—probably until a given hospital considers all-new construction.

Step Four. Is the Activity Process-Intensive or Structurally Inefficient?

This is the category that produces most of the candidates for restructuring and redeployment. Most of the problems of the current hospital operating model are directly attributable to process intensity and structural inefficiencies. Almost all functions in the hospital are provided to a broad spectrum of patients on a centralized basis. It is this centralization and the concomitant operating strategy that the new paradigm seeks to change forever. Process intensity is particularly invidious, but (like the Supreme Court's test for pornography), we should have little trouble knowing it when we see it.

- A chest X ray, involving ten minutes of clinical work, surrounded by an hour or two of structurally induced "process"
- Housekeepers with inordinate amounts of idle and on-call time (nevertheless, patients can wait an hour or more for a room to be prepared for their admission)
- Admitting clerks who are structurally unable to process more than five or six inpatients per day
- Transporters and couriers who are "busy" but in fact spend much of their time getting from assignment to assignment

Examples of process intensity are nearly endless, but some of them are not readily apparent even when the new paradigm is well understood. Sometimes an amazingly simple insight is needed to shake loose an especially entrenched deployment problem. To encourage us to look at old problems in new ways, we will return to the heroes of one of the earlier True-Life Adventures—Ms. Henderson and Mr. Wilson—as they revisit the intractable problem of productivity in the medical records department.

"Let's Try Something Different"

"I really appreciate the extra staff you approved for the department last month," Jack Wilson tells his boss, Ms. Henderson. "The backlog of loose sheets is gone, and we're now keeping up with the daily influx."

"I was a little embarrassed—even for a vice president—by the weird logic I had to use, but your three-color slides seemed to do the trick," Ms. Henderson replies. "You ought to feel lucky. Every other department the senior staff discussed at the meeting got whacked."

"If it's any consolation, I share your embarrassment. In fact, the whole idea that productivity could be up and that I still needed more staff really troubled me. I think I may have come up with a new way of looking at the whole problem. Do you have a few minutes?" Jack asks a bit sheepishly.

"Sure. But I warn you. No more staff!" Ms. Henderson answers a bit pointedly.

"Well, I started with a very basic question: what business are we in? I'm not sure I can define it precisely, but I know it isn't the loose-sheet filing business. At some basic level, we could say our business in the department is to assemble, code, archive, and analyze patient charts," Jack begins, pausing to let Ms. Henderson respond.

"So far, so good. But forgive an impertinent question. So what?"

"Something very interesting happened when I pursued that simple statement. Instead of breaking the department into several functional areas and then looking at their individual productivity numbers, I decided to use a much broader measurement of how effective we are as a whole. Here's what I mean," he continues, handing Ms. Henderson several pages of tables and charts.

"Take me through this step by step," she prompts, hoping Jack is indeed on to something.

"We have a total of eighty-five FTEs in the department. Twenty of them are devoted to transcription, and they're paid more or less by the line, so productivity isn't a big issue for us with them."

"Okay. Go on."

"Just take a leap of faith with me. Let's say we need a total of twenty-five people in the department itself to file and pull records, do analysis, and manage the whole operation. Backing out those people along with the transcriptionists still leaves forty FTEs, right?" Jack continues, building a head of steam.

"That's a lot of staff; but again, so what?" Ms. Henderson replies, uncertain that this is going anywhere.

"Well, this hospital runs a census of nearly six hundred patients with an average stay of about 6.5 days. That means we have eighty to ninety discharges per day. Do you see what I'm getting at?"

"Not yet. But that doesn't sound like an awful lot of work when you divide eighty discharges a day by forty people," Ms. Henderson responds.

"That's exactly what I'm getting at! Don't you see? If we

ignore the specific pieces of the process each of those employees does today and simply divide the number of discharges per day by forty, we find that each person would only have to complete two inpatient records per day," Jack exclaims.

"I don't know whether to laugh or cry. It isn't really that simple, is it Jack?"

"It is and it isn't. It is that easy to take this simple view of the work. It isn't so easy to follow the argument where it wants to lead us," Jack replies.

"And where is that, Jack?" she asks.

"It wants to lead us away from breaking our processes into little pieces, creating specialists to perform those little pieces, and measuring productivity by counting how many little pieces they do each month. That's how productivity can go up and yet we still require more staff," he continues, getting into a rhythm.

"I see that now. But you've only restated the problem. What's the answer?" Ms. Henderson asks, trying not to get her hopes up too high.

"I need to do some more work on it, but I'm beginning to think the answer is that we could do the work with twenty people, not forty. Four records a day ought to be a reasonable work load. But—and this is the scary part—I don't think they can do it sitting in my department. They'll have to be closer to the action. They'll need to be involved earlier in the process. They'll need access to the care givers and physicians on a regular basis. They'll need to own those four patients per day," Jack goes on, nearly running out of breath.

"So you're saying you could let twenty people go and just let the others walk the halls of the inpatient units? Quick arithmetic says it will save more than $500,000 a year. What's the catch?" Ms. Henderson asks.

"Well, we'd need to train the staff a bit more broadly than we currently do and work things out with nursing. By the way, these people wouldn't walk the halls, they would be members of a unit's team—they'd have to be, if we want them to own the *record from admission to discharge. Continuity is key. Who knows. Perhaps they could also play a role in utilization review and discharge planning. There are lots of dimensions," Jack responds, pushing the ideas one step further.*

"The training costs would be small compared to the savings. I can also see this reducing stays and improving the receivables. Jack, this is big. I want you to lead a meeting with admitting and some of my patient accounting staff to see if we can extend your 'simple' approach to some other areas," replies Ms. Henderson, clearly impressed.

"I can't believe I'm proposing something that will decimate my own department, but it seems the right thing to do for our patients both in terms of cost and service. What will I tell my people?" Jack asks, dreading the idea of layoffs.

"Look, this won't happen overnight. Your turnover rate is about 15 percent a year. When the time comes, you can tell your people we'll realize the cuts over a year or two through attrition. The gain is big enough to take a long-term perspective. Besides, we'll need some extra folks to work our way through the transition," offers Ms. Henderson.

"You know, if we push this idea across all clerical work, we might end up with a completely different organization. Maybe we'll have clerks on the units who can do it all," Jack speculates, a bit anxious about the implications of his idea.

"We might do that—and more, Jack."

On a first-cut basis, most hospital activities will emerge from this step as candidates for redeployment. Of course, not all of them will ultimately be redeployed; rather, they will be candidates when we are looking to design new operating approaches for patient care centers. In fact, even those functions that appear to be structurally efficient or less process-intensive will be examined. There is one more way in which redeploying functions can play a role in the overall restructuring, and that is addressed in the next step.

Step Five. Does the Activity Involve Deferrable Work?

Consideration of this item must be both subtle and counterintuitive, because we are seeking deferrable work that will allow us to design new, more flexible jobs on the patient care centers. Seeking such opportunities may involve looking in some unusual places in the organization.

Certain activities may be quite well organized and managed within today's operating paradigm—and there may be no reason on the surface to change things. A common example is the dietary department. Many dietary departments have become very efficient in managing their multiple missions. These departments have two primary production and delivery missions: three daily meals for inpatients and cafeteria and catering services for the staff and visitors. These two missions are often blended almost seamlessly into one operating structure and work force. Employees who assemble trays for patients in the early morning may then move on to being servers in the cafeteria line for breakfast, then retrieve carts from the inpatient units, then move back to tray assembly for the lunch service, and then help clean the equipment. The laundry may also have a well-orchestrated system for maximum productivity in sorting, washing, drying, pressing, delivery, and pickup.

Why would we want to disturb any of these well-managed functions? We would not—without good reasons. But such reasons exist. The first involves two issues that we have dealt with in depth in previous chapters: flexibility and ownership.

Departments that have made themselves efficient may have done so at the expense of flexibility in responding to patient needs. For example, red plastic bags full of dirty linen lying outside each patient's room in the midmorning are one of the hallmarks of today's operating approach. Why are they there? For the efficiency of laundry personnel. We try to change all beds in the morning so that we can get the dirty linen bagged and in the hall. Then those picking up will gather them on their rounds at, say, 11:00 A.M. With the current operating structure, this practice also complements the housekeeping department's approach to room cleaning, so we simply accept it as a part of hospital routine. When we change the housekeeping approach, we may also need to alter the linen distribution function, even if our action seems to disturb a well-run operation.

Problems with ownership and continuity may also be reasons to disturb the operations of seemingly efficient functions. Consider tray distribution to patient units and their subsequent pickup. In most hospitals, dietary personnel deliver carts full of meal trays to the patient units. The distribution function is then handed off to unit personnel who distribute the individual trays to patients, collect them, and stack them back in the cart (which is then picked up by another dietary employee). Either way we look at the process, it divorces the service provider from the customer. The dietary service loses control and ownership over meal delivery to patients; it is robbed of direct feedback from customers and control over the timeliness and friendliness of actual delivery. From the nursing staff's point of view, patient meals are simply a pain. The cart is always either early or late (it seems), patients complain about the food incessantly, and there always seem to be mistakes. Then there is the rush to pick up the trays in time to restack them in the cart before the dietary employee reappears to take it back.

But these issues, important as they are, are not really anything new; they are simply examples of potential shortcomings in the current model, shortcomings that might lead us to reexamine apparently well-run operations.

What is new here is the understanding that the jobs we design for the restructured patient care centers must have useful and effective combinations of on-demand and deferrable activities. Simply put, if we ask people to perform a wider variety of tasks, they cannot all be things that have to be performed on a strict schedule or immediately. An apt analogy here is fire fighters. Their main responsibility is a set of on-demand activities—essentially responding to alarms immediately. However, they also have considerable amounts of time that can be effectively utilized performing deferrable tasks: cooking, eating, sleeping, maintenance, grooming the Dalmatian, and so on. This same basic idea can be transplanted into the hospital environment when we redesign processes, aggregate tasks, and fashion new jobs.

The reason for moving deferrable work from a well-run area to the bedside is that we may need that work to design full jobs. The cost of the deferrable work is roughly zero. Although we may sacrifice some of the "efficiency" of a central department, the staff member to whom the work is transferred at the bedside costs us nothing. He or she would be there anyway, and we are simply using the deferrable work to make sure that employee is busy (but responsive) and to eliminate the need to interrupt continuity in the name of centralized efficiency.

On-demand work is created by patient or physician needs. It should be done as soon as possible and is either the result of a request or an event. Deferrable work has multiple dimensions. Not all tasks that are deferrable are equally so. For example, some tasks are deferrable

- *Minute to minute.* These tasks are not very helpful in job redesign. They amount to the usual task-juggling inherent in most jobs (putting one call on hold to answer another, ordering the X ray before ordering the lab work, and so on).
- *Hour to hour.* At this level, the concept of "deferrability" begins to become useful in job redesign because the staff has some real flexibility. Examples include routine linen changes and room cleaning, lab tests for some patients (assuming the existence of an on-unit lab), many documentation tasks, and care planning.
- *Shift to shift.* On especially busy days, a surprising number of tasks can fall into this time frame. Supply restocking, the posting of formal results, utilization review activities, and some routine therapies (such as gait training) are examples.
- *Day to day (or longer).* Almost every internal meeting potentially falls into this category, as do items with long (multiday) lead times, such as preadmitting work.

We should also remind ourselves that the restructuring of many centralized activities transforms a large number of tasks into the deferrable category. By decentralizing housekeeping, for instance, we remove the current requirement that patient rooms be cleaned between 7:00 A.M. and noon. Room cleaning can respond more readily to particular situations during a time span that is now sixteen hours long. The same holds true for many unit-based ancillary services such as specimen collection because we are now free from the tyranny of the centralized lab schedule. These kinds of changes are exactly what enable the new paradigm to focus on patients.

A final observation on the issue of deferrable versus on-demand work is required. Virtually every patient-originated request should be considered an on-demand request (or at most deferrable minute to minute). Most patient demands involve either personal comfort or waiting for services. Patients should not be asked to wait. This goal may seem both obvious and unrealistic. For this imperative to be operationalized, we must instill in our employees a sense of service. Nothing a patient needs is beneath the dignity of any staff member to provide. "Never, ever pass off what you can do yourself" must be the motto of the new paradigm. This alone will improve our responsiveness and flexibility.

We must also train as broadly as possible to meet on-demand requirements. We may need to train unit-based pharmacists in the rudiments of admitting, for example. It is simply unacceptable for a patient to be asked to wait fifteen minutes for the clerk to return so the patient can be admitted. Someone who can get the basic information required for treatment and orders to be executed must be available at all times. Making this happen is less a matter of the technicalities of training than it is a challenge for the culture. The culture must translate the new structure into a new set of values, incentives, and team skills that concentrates on basic patient needs.

What Is Likely to Be Redeployed?

The question of functional redeployment need not be treated as a totally indeterminate issue. Functions from hospital to hospital are similar enough to permit some educated guesses. In fact, as time goes on, it is likely that the list of redeployment candidates will become fairly standardized—at least for hospitals of a certain size (say, 150 beds and larger).

There is now sufficient experience in restructuring to suggest that many institutions may choose to examine the issue of redeployment inductively—that is, rather than going through the deployment decision tree in a linear and deductive fashion, it may be appropriate to begin with the "answer" and seek reasons *not* to redeploy certain functions. Based on our experiences to date, the following bedside deployments are likely to make sense:

- Support functions (including housekeeping, patient transportation, courier services, light maintenance, linen distribution and collection, and meal-tray distribution and collection)
- Administrative functions (including admitting, preadmission paperwork, scheduling, precertification, recertification, utilization review, chart assembly and completion, record coding, supply ordering, and inventory)
- Basic clinical functions (including phlebotomy and other specimen draws, EKG, some PT activities, and routine respiratory therapy procedures)

The deployment of the more regulated ancillary services, such as lab, X ray, and pharmacy, will show more variation from hospital to hospital and even among patient care centers within the same institution. This variation will be a reflection of differences in demand patterns, space available, technology, and local regulation.

Before leaving this topic, we should remind ourselves that the lists just given are lists of *activities*, not positions or individuals. These are simply the functions that we want to be available within the patient care centers. How we design jobs and teams around these activities is a separate issue.

The deployment of functions in the patient-focused hospital is a critical step in the restructuring process. It can also be complex and subtle. As time goes on, however, the new paradigm will begin to develop its own template for the most likely shape of functional deployment in the majority of hospitals. This will make the task somewhat easier, but it should not blind us to the fact that pat answers are antithetical to innovation. It will be a long time before we exhaust all the new and good ideas about functional deployment in the patient-focused hospital.

8

Enablers

for Change

"Enablers"—capabilities that exploit the potential of new models—operate in two directions. The first and most common are those enablers that must be in place (or developed early) to permit the paradigm shift to occur effectively. The second involves ideas that occur as a result of the paradigm shift itself and enhance its power. A perfect American analogy can be drawn from the development of the automobile. Basic roads, gas stations, rubber tire technology, and service capabilities were necessary for the car to move beyond the initial stage of its development. Once these goals were accomplished, a second wave of innovations was inspired by the automobile itself: superhighways, roadside motels, and fast food (now with drive-through service), not to mention the new technology carried on the vehicles themselves (fancy stereos, electronic engine management, and so forth). This chapter explores some of the initial enablers for patient-focused restructuring and speculates about innovations likely to be spawned by the evolution toward the new operating approach.

Documentation by Exception

Developing multidisciplinary protocols and charting by exception are the single greatest time creators involved in patient-focused restructuring. The difficulties are considerable but commensurate with the benefits. Let us review the reasons for changing today's documentation system. Figure 8.1 vividly illustrates the mess we are in.

As with so many other aspects of our current operating paradigm, no one set out to create a system this clumsy and redundant. No one asked, "How can we develop a charting system to accommodate entering vital signs in six different places?" The legal system, utilization review, and various accrediting bodies have combined with the system's own fragmentation and proclivity for detail to produce the nightmare that we now have. But we must be clear about the problem we are trying to fix. The problem is not that the chart is too thick or that there are twenty-five different medication forms. The problem is that nearly one dollar in every five that we now spend in running our hospitals is devoted to medical documentation. This is money that could be better spent delivering care to patients and better service to physicians.

We also should remind ourselves that we are unlikely to solve this problem without leaving behind our rigid operating approach. The documentation needs of patients vary dramatically but predictably. For intensive care patients, these requirements

Figure 8.1. Complexity in the Medical Record.

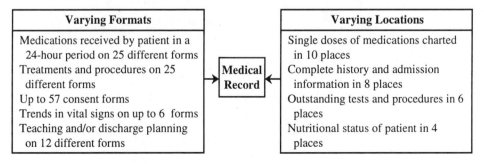

Varying Formats	Varying Locations
Medications received by patient in a 24-hour period on 25 different forms	Single doses of medications charted in 10 places
Treatments and procedures on 25 different forms	Complete history and admission information in 8 places
Up to 57 consent forms	Outstanding tests and procedures in 6 places
Trends in vital signs on up to 6 forms	Nutritional status of patient in 4 places
Teaching and/or discharge planning on 12 different forms	

(Center box: **Medical Record**)

are dominated by data, gathered repeatedly in great detail and typically showing trends over time. Outpatients, especially those seeking simple diagnostic tests, require little more than billing information. Most general surgery patients need little more than documents recording "transactions" and tracking predicted course of recovery. Medical patients are different still. Seeking one approach to these vastly varying situations is unlikely to produce anything much better than what we have today.

What therefore are the requirements of the new system that we seek? First, it must do something more than change nursing documentation. Nursing is a large part of the equation but by no means the only dimension involved. The scope of the new system must also embrace respiratory therapy, pharmacy and dietary functions, and other on-unit services. If we simply improve the nursing dimension (as large as it is), we will leave untouched all the forms and entries generated by the parade of staff that enters the patients' rooms. Furthermore, we cannot confine ourselves to "the chart." Nursing-care plans—one of the largest black holes of documentation work—must also be considered in our new system.

We therefore need a truly multidisciplinary approach to all unit-based documentation activities. Moreover, the system must be both flexible—accommodating different approaches to different sets of needs—and "open"—that is, permitting patients to move from one subsystem to another as their care needs change over the course of their stays.

Not all of these features have been worked out for all patients yet. Nevertheless, some of the early implementers of patient-focused care have made significant strides with certain groups of patients. Because of the predictability of their care requirements, surgical patients have received the most attention in the effort to streamline documentation. This area is where the benefits are easy to envision and the physicians most likely to be cooperative. In fact, these two factors are linked. For many years, surgeons have developed their own sets of preoperative and postoperative orders, sometimes sharing them directly with the nursing staff to expedite the care of their patients and minimize the need for repeated telephone calls and bedside visits. In essence, the physician would authorize the initiation of the standard orders for an uncomplicated gallbladder operation, and the nursing staff would translate these into specific transactions. In a sense, the new documentation system simply builds on this approach.

But things are never as easy as we might wish. Physicians generally resist the notion that medicine can be reduced to a "cookbook"—a favorite shibboleth. However, years of utilization review and recent federal mandates to develop practice guidelines are making resistance to protocols and care paths less strident. Furthermore, the documentation system that we seek for the patient-focused hospital provides real incentives for the physicians, unlike the other initiatives that are generally seen as intrusive and aspire to no greater end than a reduction in hospital costs. It is unlikely that the average physician will work harder and submit to what is seen as additional scrutiny just to reduce length of stay by half a day. Yet if we can offer increased continuity of care, faster turnaround of routine ancillaries, reduced documentation time, and fewer patient complaints, we will have the physician's attention and perhaps cooperation. The physician needs to see the documentation changes as part of a larger effort to improve care and service.

There are some happy stories in the effort to enlist the support and assistance of physicians. At one major academic medical center (where we might expect the greatest resistance), the chairman of orthopedics quickly agreed to the development of protocols with the sage observation, "Heck, our housestaff spend the first month of their rotation trying to figure out what our protocols are. Why don't we just tell them?"

We now know what is possible in the quest for protocols that are sufficient to permit documentation by exception—at least for procedure-based patients, such as surgery. For many of these patients (even following open-heart surgery), we can describe what should happen in four- to eight-hour blocks of time after they return from the operating room. It is also possible to describe the range of desired outcomes from these activities. For example, on the day shift of the second postoperative day for a certain surgical procedure, we might define the following activities (among others) and outcomes:

- Monitor vital signs every four hours—no fever, no respiratory symptoms
- Check wound drainage tube—no excessive drainage
- Check wound—clean; no sign of infection
- Ambulate twice for fifty paces—no dizziness or respiratory distress
- Perform CBC with differential—no indications of anemia or infection
- Return to normal diet—tolerated

And so on. If all these things have been done and the outcomes are within the desired norms, documentation can consist of a signature by a registered care giver (in addition to recording vital signs). If something has been left out or added, reasons must be documented. This simple approach obviates the need for a separate nursing-care plan and eliminates the need for the sometimes interminable prose notes that so commonly clutter today's medical records. No more remarks such as "ate dinner well" cluttering up the important information in the chart. The records will become simpler and smaller. Most impressively, the time devoted to documentation is reduced by as much as 75 percent. One particular hospital has reduced documentation time for nurses from more than two hours per nurse per day to less than fifteen minutes (for surgical patients). This saving was accomplished without the use of computer systems; a manual process was simply dramatically improved. We will return to this important point later in this chapter.

Think about what you could do in your hospital if every nurse suddenly had an hour or more per day of "free" time. This is how time is "created" in restructuring, time that can be used to absorb additional responsibilities (phlebotomy and EKG, for instance) or to enhance the personal side of the care we give.

As stated earlier, surgical patients have received the greatest attention in designing new documentation approaches. Medicine patients, especially those in the diagnostic portion of their stays, present greater challenges since their care requirements are more difficult to predict. For these patients, computer-assisted decision making may be a necessary first step in simplifying documentation. In the critical care areas, data management is the greatest challenge. Here, transducers connected to computers may help to move toward streamlining documentation. Some technology is already available for this purpose, and more will be developed. The task is still daunting, however, as the current practice of hourly assessments seems to be equal parts of making assessments and writing down the findings.

In general, we should not be discouraged. The fact that there are spectacular results for surgery patients and only embryonic efforts aimed at other patients is just what we would have predicted. When we take the time to tailor our operating approaches to special groups of patients, we need to relax our historical constraint to find one solution for all of our customers. Even if we do only one-third as well for nonsurgical patients, our efforts will have been well rewarded.

As a final note, we should consider the risk management issues raised by the protocols and documentation by exception. Here the news is uniformly good. There were concerns at first that the new approach would not satisfy the perceived requirements of litigation support and would therefore expose the hospital to additional risk. The assessments of risk management professionals seem to be quite different. The most obvious advantage of protocols is that the hospital now has very specific guidelines for how it will care for specific types of patients. Physician-to-physician variation is reduced, and the care standards are there for everyone to see. This situation is expected to make the job of defending cases easier.

The second benefit is more subtle and has to do with the

ability of the existing system to codify standards that were never intended. Let us consider a unit where the head nurse encourages the staff to make extensive notes in the chart. We will say that most nurses on the unit remark on the patients' eating habits: "ate dinner well" or "did not eat brussel sprouts." If a malpractice case should arise on this unit, the plaintiff's attorney would likely review other records of similar patients to understand both the explicit and implicit standards of care on the unit. If the attorney noticed that on the night the plaintiff died there was no entry regarding dinner consumption, a breach of an implied standard could be argued. Protocols can by and large eliminate this kind of variation.

Cross-Training

Implementing cross-training is probably not going to be as bad as you imagine. Yes, a great deal of it will be necessary, but most hospitals actually already train for the skills that will be in greatest demand. Recall that 30 percent of the work in the hospital today is clerical in nature. Another 25 to 30 percent of the jobs are scheduling, coordinating, transporting-distributing, and hotel-related activities. Just as we saw that the clinical functions of the hospital are dominated by relatively simple procedures, so too is much of the overall work load.

Perhaps the best way to illustrate this point is to look at the distribution of educational backgrounds required by the work force in the hospital. Table 8.1 shows the entry-level requirements of various positions and the percentage of the staff each represents. More than one-half of the hospital's employees come to work with no greater qualifications than a high school diploma (or some vocational training) and a willingness to learn. It is only a slight exaggeration to say that whatever these people do in their day-to-day jobs, we taught them. Many came to us with basic clerical skills, and we taught them to use the right forms, ask the right questions, and communicate with their appropriate counterparts in other departments. Housekeepers, transporters, phlebot-

Table 8.1. Formal Training of Current Nonmanagement Staff.

Education Requirements	Staff Examples	Current FTEs
Graduate degree (2–3 years post-graduate study)	• Pharmacists	31
Bachelor's degree (3–4 years study)	• Senior medical technologists • Medical technologists • Education specialists	91
	• Registered nurses (including admitting and emergency room specialists)	587
Associate degree or technical school certificate (1.5–2 years)	• Radiological technicians • Respiratory therapists • Cardiovascular technicians	105
	• Licensed practical nurses	122
Some technical or trade school training (6 months–1 year)	• Surgical technicians • Medical transcriptionists • Medical records coder-abstractors • Skilled maintenance tradesmen	135
High school diploma or less	• Unit coordinators • Nursing assistants • Environmental service aides • Pharmacy technicians • Lab assistants and clerks • EKG technicians • Dietetics assistants • Phlebotomists	900
	Total	1,971

omists, laundry workers, couriers, and even some technical workers are largely staff members trained by the hospital through some combination of more formal instruction and on-the-job training. Nurses, technologists, and other professionals (excluding managers) make up less than 25 percent of all hospital employees.

This fact is especially important because the skills that dominate the work today are precisely those we are going to be teaching most extensively in the patient-focused hospital. For every nurse who may also be trained to perform a basic battery of lab tests (where this is legal), we will probably be training ten staff members to perform a broader assortment of clerical or support tasks. Furthermore, as we look to extend the capability of employees to perform certain basic clinical functions (say, phlebotomy and EKG), we will by and large be working with people who are already clinically focused.

With this perspective, the cross-training hurdle should be manageable for most hospitals. Yes, it may require some increased educational resources, but it does not entail commissioning every hospital as a school of allied health sciences. Where cross-training for certain lab and X ray work is permitted, those departments themselves are likely to be the source of the curriculum and the teaching resources. Community colleges may also play a growing role in preparing the health care workers of the future—combining several narrow areas of preparation into multidimensional skills. Forward-thinking hospitals will work with them to fashion their curricula and provide a reliable source of better-paying jobs for the graduates. We should also expect to see the further development of computer-assisted and interactive training technologies.

The Real Training Challenge

The conceptual and technical challenges of the paradigm of patient-focused care are significant, but as time goes on we will see more and more of them conquered. Almost predictably, they will themselves become the components of a new canon, accepted and applied with decreasing variation among institutions. Such is the fate of any sound model.

The enduring legacy of patient-focused care is likely to be its impact on the dimension of operations that is most difficult to change: organizational culture. Long after our new structures and systems have been superseded by something even better, the sea change in hospital culture will survive—*if* we change it today and continue to reinforce the values and meaning of patient-focused care over the longer term.

The greatest challenge of any new paradigm (and this one in particular) is to change the way people act and the way they *think*. The structural changes that we implement will almost force our employees to change the way they act, but that is not sufficient. Clear leadership is needed that will also change the way they feel about their work. Fixing the operating structure of a 400-bed hospital is the easy part. Winning over the hearts and minds of two thousand employees is the hard part.

To illustrate the kind of change that is required and the power that it represents, let us consider the experience of a clerical employee at a large East Coast hospital. Before the restructuring at this hospital, she had been an admitting clerk. She met many patients each day and completed the necessary paperwork for their admission. She was then trained to work on a new patient care center, with duties including admissions, unit-based clerical work, utilization review, and some medical records activities. What is moving about her experience with patient-focused care is her changed motivation for doing the work well. In the old world, she did her job well to keep her boss happy. In her new job, she works carefully and well because if she does not, the patients will get hassled by their insurance companies and the hospital business office. She knows from personal experience how upsetting this can be and how frustrating it is to deal with the faceless bureaucracy. She now has control over enough of the patient's paperwork that she herself can assure its accuracy and completeness. Furthermore, she feels an intense personal ownership of the work on the patient's behalf. This is a patient-focused employee, and we need many more like her.

Accomplishing this cultural transformation and maintaining it are the enduring challenges of the patient-focused hospital. There is no recipe and never will be. There are, however, some basic components of the transformation. They are practical and deceptively simple. The first step, of course, is the creation of an operating structure (and jobs within it) that makes patient-focused care possible and that puts employees close enough to the total care process that a sense of ownership is even a possibility. But that is clearly not enough. The hospital's staff—all of it, from executives to the front line—must know and embrace the goals and values of the new paradigm. This process begins with frequent communication and reinforcement, tailored to specific groups of employees, during the design and early implementation phase. Team skills must be taught as an integral part of the training curriculum. Retraining must include managers, because nothing will short-circuit the effort faster than managers who live in the old world and thwart the initiatives of the newly empowered work force. Continuous quality improvement must be instituted to maintain the momentum and close the customer-service loop.

Compensation Systems

The present compensation systems are fitting reflections of our current operating strategy and structure. We are most comfortable with systems that reward increasing specialization and technical skills. Furthermore, to the extent that productivity enters into the equation, we are most likely to measure it by the number of similar or identical tasks performed per unit of time. Status is conferred by the extent to which the system recognizes the uniqueness of a given staff member's educational background and technical qualifications. The system has been only too happy to accommodate this minute differentiation; recall that it is common for one-half of the positions (titles) in a hospital to held by just one incumbent. Performance bonuses and incentive compensation are rare below the management level, probably because individual contributions to overall performance by narrowly focused staff are so hard to measure.

Compensation systems for patient-focused hospitals are still in their early stages of development. Nonetheless, the long-term goals for such systems are clear. We want fewer positions rather than more (one hospital has the goal of defining only forty different jobs after restructuring); the positions should be more broadly defined; they should be capable of rewarding breadth, not just depth; they should encourage personal growth and ownership of patients; and they should include appropriate incentives.

In all likelihood, our new work force will be compensated more per person because we will demand more from job performance than we now do. Many approaches are likely to emerge that meet these criteria.

A background note on the evolution of new compensation systems may be useful. The very first institutions to attempt patient-focused restructuring approached the initiative as experiment. It was by no means clear that the new model would survive its initial test, and it was therefore necessary to encourage participation and minimize the personal risk assumed by the staff members who volunteered to participate. A range of approaches was used—all with the guarantee of being able to return to one's old position without penalty, either because the experiment failed or because the staff member could not adapt. The results of these three approaches are useful as we move forward and consider the attitudes toward change and the need for incentives.

One hospital offered a flat 10 percent increase in compensation for the duration of training and the "pilot" phase of the effort. The need for longer-term changes would be addressed at the conclusion of the six-month trial period. Another hospital offered a $1,000 bonus payment, provided in two parts. Each staff member would receive $500 at the successful conclusion of the cross-training classes. The other $500 would be paid if the pilot was deemed a success at the end of six months (with measures and parameters laid out in advance). The third hospital offered no financial incentives at all.

Surprisingly, there was little difference in the experiences of these institutions. Recruitment of staff members was not remarkably easier or harder under the different circumstances, and all three hospitals reported employee turnover rates well below those of their institutions as a whole. Very few participants dropped out (or were dropped) during the training period. These experiences seem to support recent studies of cross-training that have found that financial incentives are not the primary motivators of staff in the acquisition of new skills. The challenge and the variety of the work itself appear to be the major forces at work.

Whether this finding will be true for most hospital employees or will be sustained over time remains to be seen.

One particular hospital, though, has invested a good deal of time in developing a new compensation approach for employees in a patient-focused environment. The system focuses initially on the staff assigned to bedside care on a patient care center (this classification, by the way, embraces roughly 75 percent of the staff members on the unit). All of these employees carry one title and one classification in the compensation system: multiskilled practitioner. They have this title regardless of their background and role—nursing assistants, respiratory therapists, radiology technologists, or registered nurses. The established pay range for this new classification is from about $5.00 per hour to $25.00 per hour. How much people earn is roughly proportional to their answer to the question, "What can you do?" Yes, there are educational gates within the point range, but there is also considerable pay mobility. For example, if employees can clean floors, change beds, and transport patients, they might earn $5.00 per hour. However, if they add the skills of ambulating patients, checking vital signs, and performing phlebotomy, their pay might rise to $6.75 per hour. Many of the skills that can be added are available through in-service or on-the-job training. At the top of the range, an RN who is capable of caring for the center's full range of patients (say, urology, general surgery, orthopedics, and ENT) and who can lead teams and teach staff in all those areas may earn $25.00 per hour—potentially 15 percent more than the manager to whom that person reports. This is a true clinical ladder.

One final aspect of such compensation systems merits attention. Unions are present in many hospitals (in addition to the many guilds with which we deal whose mandates come from state legislation or accreditation standards). Since most unions are "trade" organizations, they mirror (and complicate) the existing compartmentalization and specialization of our hospitals. We might also predict that they would be openly hostile to any restructuring efforts that seek to blur distinctions between jobs. However, though the unions are by no means enthusiastic supporters, there are signs of hope. Upon hearing about patient-focused restructuring for the first time, several leaders of national unions had a very curious reaction—and one that should give every hospital administrator pause. They found much to like about the concepts but felt that the greatest obstacle to implementation would be that management would never agree to let employees work in self-directed teams with real authority to solve problems on the front lines. The leaders had already understood one of the problems that the new paradigm seeks to remedy: that complex, parallel, and vertical hierarchies are the enemies of both customer service and employee job satisfaction. The union leaders especially liked the opportunities for growth, increased wages, and job security that would result from the restructuring and appropriate compensation and training programs.

This attitude, combined with recent experiences at specific hospitals, shows there is hope for the new order, even in institutions that are basically union shops. Restructuring has been accomplished in other U. S. industries that are highly unionized, but these often had convincing arguments to get the unions to the bargaining table. The industries (such as steel and the automakers) could cite declines in earnings and stock prices and could demonstrate that the world market simply would not pay the prices required by the costs of their traditional operating structures. They could translate this into a believable scenario: "We can either have five hundred jobs at this factory or we can have zero jobs, but we cannot have eight hundred jobs." Their very existence was at issue. Few hospitals can credibly make this claim. As hospitals with unions move towards patient-focused care, they are likely to bring the unions into the process early and make them partners in a long-term effort to improve patient care, enhance the quality of work life, and build sustainable jobs for the future.

Information Systems

Hospital information systems currently do exactly what we ask of them. Like the systems in any other industry, they simply mirror and reinforce the operating structures within which they function. They are true enablers of whatever paradigm that they seek to serve.

For hospitals, this means that our systems are miracles of transaction processing. Their mission is to generate line-item bills, often for a dizzying array of requirements by various third-party payers. The general ledger is highly automated, as are payroll, accounts receivable, and accounts payable. And to the extent that the same channels that receive orders for service can report results, that is helpful too. But make no mistake about it, the typical hospital information system of today is all about counting things and either charging for them or paying for them. By and large, clinical applications are either afterthoughts or the province of turnkey subsystems (self-contained systems for specific departments) that piggyback as best they can.

A recent survey seems to imply that this focus is changing. It reports that the fastest-growing segment of the hospital information systems business is clinical applications. Unfortunately, a close reading of the footnotes reveals that the bulk of these are in fact order-entry capabilities. Nothing more is being changed than the location of the cash register within the hospital. Future innovations will have to do something meaningful with the form and functionality of such bedside hardware.

Computers will not lead the patient-focused care revolution; they will follow it. This is the way it should be. Too many managers behave like the beleaguered commuter who buys a Porsche thinking that it will shorten the drive to and from the office. Unfortunately, the speed potential of this new toy is thwarted by overall traffic volume and the road system itself. Computers are the same in a sense. Buying a newer, faster model cannot improve the operating structure, only the execution of transactions within the parameters of that structure. In fact, when systems try to do more, they are usually stymied by the existing paradigm and produce nothing but frustration and disillusionment. Computers in hospitals today do a reasonably good job of handling the staggering volume of transactions that the structure produces. Future innovations will come from building information systems tailored to the new operating system.

Even modest investments in seemingly patient-focused technologies may be misguided unless they are explicitly understood to be experimental or educational. For example, let us think back to the hospital that reduced nursing documentation time from two hours per nurse per day to less than fifteen minutes. Recall also that this feat was accomplished purely through manual systems improvements (protocols and documentation by exception). This hospital was smart. Its management realized there would be very little incremental benefit from spending millions on a computer system that would reduce the time required from fifteen minutes to ten. Clearly, any new computer system that purports to revolutionize medical documentation will have to do something far more dramatic to justify its price.

The Future Information System

A patient-focused information system does not exist as of this writing. Nevertheless, it is possible to speculate on the general architecture and features that such a system is likely to have. Its basic goal should be to invert today's approach. Current systems are forced to assist in managing the hospital "from the bill in." Patient-focused systems will enable the hospital of the future to be managed "from the bed out." Rather than using computers to manage transactions (with patient care management being an afterthought at best), we can capitalize on the concentration of resources at the bedside to manage both care and the business side of the enterprise. Pulling all the concepts, imperatives, and implications together, the patient-focused information system is likely to be

- Composed of building blocks, discrete systems tailored to the operating environments of the patient care centers. There may be as many as five or six of these basic operating environments and related building blocks. As discussed earlier, these could be those that are short stay and transaction-intensive

(for example, surgery), data management–intensive (critical
care), decision support–intensive (medical diagnostic), low
intensity (longer stay–convalescent), and minimal-problem
(routine outpatient).

- Served by sophisticated data management hardware that permits patients to move easily between care environments when
  necessary.
- Eventually linked to other care sites, such as doctors' offices,
  primary care centers, diagnostic facilities, home health providers, and (perhaps some day) patients' homes.
- Adept at using new direct-input devices and transducers to
  reduce the need to transcribe data. The new system will not
  simply substitute writing in the record with typing on the
  computer.
- Capable of using primarily clinical activity data to manage
  the patient care center. For example, staff planning and even
  billing could be readily generated based on what was happening at the bedside (this is part of the meaning of managing
  from the "bedside out").

How might a system such as this actually work on a patient
care center? Let us consider a surgical patient care center where
virtually all of the patients' care is driven by protocols (in the
computer), and charting is done by exception against those protocols. Much of the basic admitting data may be gathered by the
physicians in their offices. The bed, the care team, and the operating room can all be scheduled simultaneously with one call or
computer transaction. As care is delivered to the patients by their
teams, the system is constantly updated. Teams that are in trouble
with their work loads can be identified by the manager of the
center almost immediately, and help can be dispatched. Further,
if a patient is not ambulated on a given day shift, the system will
alert the manager not because the care team has made a mistake
but because it may mean that this patient will not go home as
planned. This could generate a series of actions involving utiliza-

tion review and revisions of the incoming patients' assignments to care teams later in the week. If a patient's condition has worsened and a transfer to critical care is necessary, the system would translate all the information to date into a form compatible with the data management system in use in the intensive care environment. Further, just as care can be delivered by protocol and charted by exception, order entry and charging can also be accomplished almost invisibly by the system.

It should also be noted that the patient care centers of the future will manage their business quite differently than they do now. Today we (and our computers) are obsessed with counting things—admissions, units of service, charges, and the like. We are absolutely addicted to such numbers, even if we cannot really manage what we are counting. The patient care centers of the future—since they contain 70 to 80 percent of their patients' costs—will be managed less like factories and more like cruise ships. Once a cruise ship leaves port, the majority of its costs are fixed. Staff members cannot be laid off at sea. Further, most cruise ships include meals (but not drinks) and entertainment in a fixed price. Why? Because within reasonable bounds, these items are not critical to profitability and because the cost of keeping track of precisely what each passenger eats and which shows are attended simply is not worth the trouble. Most of the cost is tied up in the ship itself: its fuel consumption, dock fees, and, of course, the fixed staff for the voyage.

Patient care centers will manage themselves in a similar way. Within reasonable limits, the capital investment and the staffing are fixed. Furthermore, variations in the consumption of routine supplies, food, and even unit-based ancillary tests are not a major concern. A $100 catheter (like drinks on the cruise ship) may warrant a separate charge (and the infrastructure that goes along with it). A trip to the operating room or the CAT scanner might be treated like ports of call for the patient and might generate separate charges. In this environment, you can see why counting the number of CBCs performed would be a poor use of management time and attention. The staff required to draw the sample and run the test is fixed, the machine is always there, and the reagent-solution cost is too small to worry about. We might be concerned about the number of CBCs because of unnecessary discomfort for the patient. This understanding will require a whole new mindset for management.

Computer Systems During the Transition

Virtually every hospital today has a computer system—at least for accounting, its general ledger, and admitting-discharge-transfer functions. Many computers are quite new, fast, expensive, and sophisticated. What should we do with our systems strategy until the patient-focused care systems hit the market (at least two years from now)? The best counsel on this question has three aspects: adaptation, investment, and incremental functionality.

Much like the Hippocratic oath, the first rule of living in the computer limbo between paradigms is Do No Harm. At the very least, we must make certain that concern over today's computer does not get in the way of patient-focused restructuring (either as a reason not to begin the journey or as an obstacle to meaningful implementation). Many of the current systems can be adapted and even turbocharged to be more compatible with the new operating environment. For example, many existing systems make order entry and charging rather difficult; the routines are clearly designed for use by clerks, not care givers. The drill goes something like this. We tell the machine who we are, who the patient is, what we want to do (order a procedure, say), and what sort of procedure we wish (X ray, hematology, chemistry, and so forth). Then we choose the procedure from a series of screens listing the possibilities in alphabetical order. It is not a huge task to tailor this clumsy process for care givers and specific patient types. With computers in every room and order entry about the only thing we use them for, the process can be streamlined. The first screen to appear could simply list the procedures most likely to be ordered (by frequency distribution) for that sort of patient. For 80 percent or so of procedures, ordering could be as simple as entering an authorization code and touching an item on the first screen once with a light pen. This procedure may not be fully patient-focused perhaps, but it is better than the current one.

Now is not the time to spend major amounts of capital on new information systems that serve the old order. If you are not fully committed to a new system purchase, defer it. If you are already in the midst of an installation, make the best of it. At least take the opportunity to cable every patient room in the hospital and try to streamline whatever functions you can so that care givers can use them efficiently. Explore options to pare the system down to its accounting features, since we are likely to need that functionality for a good many years to come.

There are some judicious investments that may make sense for hospitals moving towards patient-focused care. Portable and miniaturized technologies, such as hand-held blood analyzers, will be a fact of life in the future. Gaining experience with these devices and putting them in the hands of a variety of care givers will probably be effort well spent. Technologies that foster a decentralized approach to information handling are also of interest. Bedside data devices and digital radiography fall into this category. Some of these technologies will not pay for themselves in the current operating structure. The desire to pursue their acquisition will probably need to be based on a belief that these are important technologies of the future and therefore merit evaluation and experimentation today. Be cautious, though, because these developments are not going to fix the problems of today.

Facilities

Patient-focused restructuring is not exclusively a rich organization's toy. Some of the early pioneers did invest considerably in renovating their facilities and equipping their new patient care centers, but they were generally driven by a desire to give the brand-new concepts the best possible chances for success. Further, many of the renovation costs were not incremental but represented modest increases over the amount of money that most hospitals would spend every five to seven years to upgrade and modernize existing patient care units. The equipment redeployment was also done to test the concepts in depth. In addition, the hospitals did not seek more focused technological solutions for the patient care centers—that is, whatever machines were in use, say, in the laboratory for a given test, were duplicated in the unit-based mini-labs. This approach will change over time as more experience is gained and more technology is designed for small-volume applications.

With this background in mind, we can draw some early conclusions about the opportunities and constraints inherent in the facilities dimension of patient-focused care. The first lesson (drawn from experience, not extensive analysis) is that the facility dimension is at most the last 25 percent of the patient-focused opportunity, not the first 75 percent. This conclusion comes from looking at two radically different facility configurations at two of the pioneering institutions. One, a large community hospital, had a physical plant accommodating 120 or so beds on one floor. Another, an academic medical center, placed its 30-bed pilot unit in a cylindrical building. The community hospital established a very large patient care center on three wings of one floor. The teaching hospital's unit was spread across two contiguous floors of only fifteen beds each. The good news is that the results from both facilities were consistently encouraging. Process redesign, decentralization, and cross-trained teams appear to be the source of most benefits.

The second lesson is that nominal facility changes—rather than wholesale renovation—can further enable the patient-focused transformation. There is a fairly short list of necessary items: patient servers in the rooms, computers accessible to care givers (either in all rooms or in zones), and some private space for patients and families during the admitting and financial counseling process. All of this can be accomplished without any net additional space since the current nursing station can be reduced in size to reflect the fact that it will no longer be the major work site and meeting place for the unit.

For institutions that decide to redeploy ancillaries (lab, X

ray, and pharmacy), the space challenge and investment requirement will be greater. Although none of these consumes a great
deal of room (especially if portable X rays are the mode), they
generally require space that is hard to find. In addition, a capital
investment on the order of $500,000 may be required. This is
likely to be necessary in the long run, and it does not require a
great leap of financial faith to justify it; we need only save the
equivalent of two fully loaded FTEs somewhere in the hospital
to repay such an investment. For the hospitals that will still consider this sum a major obstacle, it is becoming clear that there
are alternatives to the sequential rollout of pilot projects (each
custom-made before start-up). The facility changes and ancillary
redeployment could come in a second or third wave of the implementation initiatives. The initial wave, as mentioned before, could
take the form of redesigning and redeploying basic bundles of
support services and clerical activities. These actions require little
in the way of capital investment and are likely to generate near-
term savings to finance further patient-focused enhancements.

There are at least three hospitals today that are redesigning
their facilities from scratch using patient-focused care concepts.
This process is both exciting and a bit scary. The designs are not
set in stone, but some of the early ideas are intriguing. Flexibility
is one overriding design imperative. Some hospitals are considering making a considerable portion of their beds ICU-capable.
This approach will allow for any further trends toward hospitals'
becoming intensive care centers and will even permit rethinking
our current approach to staging care. In the name of continuity,
patient-focused hospitals may choose to move technology and
staffing resources to patients as they get sicker (and reduce them
as their conditions improve), rather than the current practice of
bouncing the patient from unit to unit. Flexibility is also para-
mount in the design of central functions.

Our current architectural paradigm of the patient care
"tower" sitting atop the diagnostic and support "pancake" will
be revised. Hospitals are likely to become more horizontal in
their conception. Larger patient care centers will be housed on

floors of eighty beds or more wherever possible. Surgical suites may be located on the same level as surgical beds. For hospitals with the option, the offices of physicians could be attached at the same level as the services that they need most often (for example, a single level of the complex might house surgeons' offices, inpatient surgery beds, and multipurpose surgical suites). We can even imagine asking the question, "Can some inpatient rooms be made capable of surgery?" There are probably good reasons why this is not possible, but the idea of LDRP-type rooms for certain patients is intriguing. Just consider all the expensive space in the operating and recovery rooms that sits idle 50 to 65 percent of the time; then consider the potential for improved continuity of care for the patients.

Smaller hospitals have the opportunity to explore the idea of a one-story building (or at least it will seem one story to the customer). Much like Disney World, any necessary second level could be below the main customer areas and invisible to patients. A one-level operation could potentially simplify ancillary deployment decisions because central services could be within the line of sight for patients and care givers. Furthermore, the traffic jams and service delays produced by elevators could be all but eliminated.

New facilities would permit the exploration of previously deferred deployment decisions. Areas like dietary have received little attention to date because of the investments they represent and the difficulty of squeezing them onto today's patient care floors. We can look for some surprising developments and innovations in the years ahead.

Technology—especially information highways—will be accommodated by the design. In addition, the design must make changes in technology relatively easy to adopt.

Although no numbers are currently available, some informed speculation on capital costs is possible. An early investigation into this issue was conducted by Llewelyn•Davies of London several years ago. Its model suggests that the patient-focused hospital will require more capital equipment but less overall space (bricks and mortar). The estimate of the net effect would be an 11 percent reduction in total capital costs when compared to a traditional hospital design. Even if this figure is only half right, the impact (especially when combined with operational savings) would be stunning indeed.

Every function and activity in the hospital will eventually need to evolve its own enablers of patient-focused care. Their details are still being explored and developed. This chapter has reviewed several major initiatives that affect the overall operation and organizational transformation. The smaller scale and more focused enablers that emerge for individual hospital activities will be one of the more exciting arenas of innovation in the months and years ahead.

9

Does It Work?

The short answer to the question of whether patient-focused care works is yes. We should probably pursue this issue at greater length, however. Virtually all of the hospitals that have implemented this approach to care began with a set of parameters to be measured as the program proceeded. These included clinical factors, satisfaction levels, utilization, service performance, and cost. This chapter addresses some of the early results in each of these areas, beginning with their expected outcomes. Some of them were especially encouraging in their magnitude, and some of the benefits, even if expected, were pleasant surprises indeed. The results are generally presented in narrative form rather than in tables and charts; moreover, the samples in some cases are too small to permit any elegant significance testing. Although some of the outcomes could be dismissed as anecdotal, reliance on this kind of information is inevitable when we are changing paradigms in the real world as opposed to a controlled, laboratory environment. Faith, common sense, and a bit of skepticism are probably the best tools for evaluating the results so far.

Background

We must keep in mind that all of the results come from institutions that have embarked on the "pilot" implementation path. They chose to test the concepts in depth for a subset of the patient population in order to answer two questions: will this work and will we kill anybody? To test the new approach in all its dimensions (including ancillary redeployment), a full, working unit was needed but it could be small. In fact, the first pilot project opened its doors with twenty staff and one patient! The work load for the teams was then gradually increased to determine the appropriate spans of care under the new model.

Everyone today wants to know whether this new paradigm actually saves money, but that was not the highest-priority question for the original implementers. Implicitly, they adopted a true TQM approach. Using this method, reduced cost is not a goal of the process but rather an outcome of doing the process right. Costs would essentially take care of themselves—by decreasing either in absolute magnitude or in cost per unit (because of increased demand). Admittedly, many of these hospitals were very successful and could indulge in the luxury of this point of view (perhaps that contributed to their past success as well). But just as importantly, they realized that they were beginning a multiyear journey. To get the support of the work force, several hospitals guaranteed that no employee would be laid off because of the restructuring. The long time line would permit attrition to take care of any necessary reductions, and cross-training could accommodate any dislocations of staff across departments and functions.

But the issue of cost remains—especially when we realize that the sequential implementation of pilot projects is not only a lengthy process but one that moves savings well into the future. The savings are realized for the most part by reducing and restructuring central departments, actions that are only possible after a majority of the patient units have been restructured. Nevertheless, more and more hospitals today are evaluating patient-focused care primarily (or at least initially) on the cost dimension. Many of these institutions are thus impatient for definitive cost information, preferably from hospitals that have completed the transformation. Unfortunately, audited financials are not available, and no hospital to date has completed full implementation.

The service that the pioneering hospitals have performed for our field is answering the most common key questions about patient-focused care: will it work? and will we kill anybody? The important question now is how do we best implement the concepts? The latest development in this area is that there does appear to be an implementation approach that is faster than pilot projects and moves the cost savings closer to the beginning of the process. Over the next year or so, a number of hospitals will be implementing patient-focused care horizontally—that is, instead of restructuring everything that they do for a subset of patients, they will be restructuring several bundles of functions hospitalwide. This system has the advantage of affecting patients and staff throughout the hospital at a fairly early stage in the process. Furthermore, the positions that are restructured and redeployed (clerks, general support workers, and middle management) are those that generate a disproportionate percentage of potential savings. Further implementation then proceeds in "waves" until all functions have been addressed and patients reaggregated.

We all look to the months and years ahead, which will provide exciting information about the advantages and challenges of full implementation. In the meantime, the results from early implementers have been no less interesting and impressive.

Service Factors

Everyone involved in the initial round of implementation agreed that dramatically improved service performance should be an immediate benefit of the patient-focused care concepts. These factors, unlike cost issues, could be demonstrated in a micro environment. Furthermore, everyone would know immediately if reductions in process complexity and improvements in continuity were of the order of magnitude expected.

In some regards, service performance is a tricky thing to measure. Personal perspective is critical. A recent article presented a vivid example of the importance of one's particular point of view in assessing service. The researchers were interested in studying response times when patients push their nurse call buttons. The answer proved elusive. Nurses deemed a call answered when they determined the nature of the patient's request. Patients, quite understandably, deemed their call answered when their need was met. Naturally, nurses reported much faster response times than did their customers. This story belongs somewhere in the curriculum of every health care worker's education or hospital orientation.

Similar examples are not hard to find. On the one hand, the lab will tell you that the average sample is analyzed within thirty minutes of its arrival in the lab. On the other, the attending physician will tell you that the turnaround time was fourteen hours, since the system required that a routine test be ordered the evening before for results by 10:00 A.M. the next day. The pharmacy processes a new drug order in about thirty minutes, but the time from the physician's order until the drug is administered is more likely to be four hours.

In the patient-focused care world, we have to be especially careful about how we measure service levels. Since we do not have a uniform operating approach, there will not be large quantities of ancillary work processed simultaneously and uniformly. In a sense, we have a just-in-time system. Some chest films, say, will be performed within a few minutes of the order, and others may be performed seven hours later. Yet both will be done precisely when they are needed. By the way, those that are performed immediately are not necessarily "stat" in the traditional sense, they are simply tests performed to accommodate the particular needs of an attending physician and a patient. Flexibility is the mode of operations. By being close enough to both doctors and patients, unit-based staff members can respond as needed, prioritize, and even defer some of their work. For example, bed changes no longer have to be squeezed into a four-hour window of time in the morning; they can be spread out across two shifts and be responsive to patient schedules and preferences.

The first indication that the patient-focused care concepts can live up to their potential is the significant reduction in process complexity for unit-based services. The range of processes includes both ancillary and administrative services.

Unit-based radiology procedures show some of the most dramatic improvements. Recall that a chest film in today's centralized environment usually entails forty or more steps, about two hours of process time, and perhaps as many as ten to twelve different employees. On the new patient care centers, work steps are cut by 50 percent or more and involve one to three people, and the work time is generally less than twenty minutes. Although the film is still read by a centralized radiologist, the attending physician can view the film before it is sent out and make a near-term care decision. Just as importantly, the patient is not wheeled through the hospital and subjected to the possibility of long waits at each end of the process. Nor is the patient unavailable for one to two hours. He or she can therefore receive other treatments (or just enjoy peace and quiet).

The admitting process has also shown major improvements—not just in waiting and processing time but also in the speed with which care givers can actually initiate the physicians' orders. For unit-based admissions, patients do not have to wait. Furthermore, for scheduled admissions, much of the work has been completed by phone in advance by a clerk who is on the unit and with the patient throughout the stay. One hospital reports that the initiation of admitting orders (food, drugs, tests, and so forth) in its current operating environment has often required three to five hours. For many patients, this lag has meant delays in receiving palliative drugs or something as simple as a cold drink or a snack. On the new care centers, the time required for admitting has been reduced to a matter of minutes after the patient's arrival.

Another dimension of perceived improvements in service—one unintended but welcome—should be highlighted here. Most hospitals that have implemented patient-focused care have provided patient servers in the room, and the medical record is now kept there. By and large, physicians are not accustomed to this system and generally resist such a change. Their typical mode of operation today is to go to the nursing station, find their patients' records, review them, and only then go to visit the patients on rounds. They believe this is an efficient use of their time and presents their best possible face to their patients ("The doctor knew all about my condition and progress before walking into my room!"). The physicians were reluctant to appear uninformed in front of their patients by reviewing the charts in the rooms, and they also feared that they would spend more time on the unit by extending the obligatory exchange of pleasantries with each patient. Once physicians were convinced to try the new system, a strange thing happened. First, the physicians reported that the new system did not result in any loss of efficiency in their rounds; the time spent was about the same. At the same time, the patients perceived that their doctors spent more time with them. As one surgeon put it, "That perception will probably save me one lawsuit over the next few years."

Neither this section nor this book would be complete without the following story, which illustrates both the need to customize the operating approach and the wisdom of empowering employees on the front lines of patient care. The story concerns a hospital in a state where cross-training for routine lab work is permissible.

Upon their arrival at the new surgical patient care center, all bedside staff members were trained by the lab to perform some simple chemistry and hematology studies (those most frequently needed by their patients). It was expected that each team would perform its own lab work throughout the day. Yet many of the surgeons never seemed to break their old habit of ordering tests the night before and wanting to see the results on their early morning rounds. What happened, of course, was a major traffic jam outside the unit's minilab each morning. Care givers would stand in line to do their tests, and the problem was compounded by the required log-on–log-off procedures for each new operator of each machine.

The patient care center team reacted quickly and developed an elegantly simple solution. One care giver (a former nursing assistant, in fact) was designated to perform all the morning lab work. She would come in an hour or so before her normal shift began and run all the tests ordered for the morning rounds. She would then join her team for a normal day's work as a multiskilled care giver. For the balance of the day, the other care givers would run their lab work themselves on an as-needed basis. Since 60 percent or so of the daily lab work was done in the early morning, the traffic jams never reappeared because the teams were running just a few tests scattered throughout the day. The hospital is still hoping to change the surgeons' behavior so that the patients can sleep late, but for the moment the unit has arrived at its own patient-focused solution to current demand patterns.

Clinical Factors

The problems addressed at the original hospitals were related to service and cost, not clinical outcomes (these were already outstanding). Because of this fact, the expectations for clinical performance were only that it should not be worse than today. Nevertheless, the results were overwhelmingly positive, and some were unexpected.

In the category of measures that could not be worse than today, the hospitals evaluated primarily negative outcomes.

- *Readmission for the same diagnosis or postsurgical complications and infections.* These areas all showed slight declines, although the small sample size probably only justifies the conclusion that performance was at least as good as it was previously.
- *Medication errors.* Though our expectation was modest ("no worse"), the outcomes here were significantly improved. Several units not only reported declines, but their rates were

now the best in the hospital. Clearly, the presence of pharmacists on the units and the improved continuity of care paid dividends.

- *Patient "incidents."* These are occurrences (like falls or errors) that require the filling out of a report for risk management purposes. Although not all hospitals tracked the number of incidents, those that did reported declines. They also reported that patients seemed better oriented to their environment and less confused (an admittedly subjective assessment). They attributed this improvement to greater continuity of care (fewer unfamiliar faces).
- *Death rates.* Here again, the relative smallness of the sample size limits its significance, but there was no evidence that the rates had changed.

In addition to these "default" measurements and assessments, other clinical factors were studied and compared to those of the previous order. Chief among these were utilization measures: average length of stay (ALOS) and ancillary consumption. In the case of ALOS, we had hopes that it would grow shorter but would have been satisfied with no change. Ancillary consumption was a different matter. There were skeptics who believed that unit-based X ray and laboratory-use rates would increase since their availability and speed would make "abuse" even more attractive. No increase would have been a victory; a decline seemed too much to hope for. Once again, results exceeded expectations.

Average length of stay declined 5 to 15 percent for all surgical populations studied. An initial evaluation attributed most of the decline to fairly standardized protocols of care, and these were clearly a contributing factor; the variations in care from doctor to doctor were now more concentrated around the mean. However, even a hospital that did not initially implement protocols noticed a reduction. Something else was at work. At one hospital, a study showed that patients on the new unit had fewer postoperative temperature spikes than other patients and that these spikes were less severe and of shorter duration. The causality is not absolutely certain, but a change in respiratory care is suspected to be helping. Today we generally wait for a patient to exhibit respiratory symptoms and then launch a series of tests and treatments (chest films, lab tests, antibiotics, and respiratory therapy). The new approach tends to use respiratory interventions prophylactically. This, and perhaps more aggressive and frequent ambulation, are likely contributors to the reduced lengths of stay.

Consumption of unit-based ancillary services was down significantly. As mentioned in an earlier chapter, the unit-based services—particularly the lab—can be used more judiciously by the attending staff members. Rapid response and even the sequencing of tests enable them to be more selective in their ordering patterns; they know that the next test is only minutes away if necessary, not hours in the future.

Measures of clinical quality and outcomes will receive much more attention and study as patient-focused care is initiated in more hospitals. We have probably only scratched the surface of this dimension. We are likely to see some hospitals combine these concepts with Planetree-like models of design and interaction. (Planetree, located in San Francisco, is well-known in the field for its innovations in hospital design and patient participation in care.) This could be an especially interesting and powerful approach, with opportunities for in-depth studies of outcomes and perceptions of quality. We will also see broader definitions of what is considered clinical. For example, let us consider the transportation of patients to and from the operating rooms. Under the patient-focused paradigm, this could be considered a clinical transaction—taking an anxious patient to a scary place and returning this disoriented patient to the floor. Most hospitals today seem to think it is just fine to have these tasks performed by a stranger earning minimum wage. Patient-focused hospitals insist this is important clinical work to be performed by a skilled and familiar care giver. These changes in perspective merit an examination of their impact on patient perceptions and outcomes.

Value Added—Changes in Where the Money Goes

One of the key objectives of patient-focused care is to change the value-added structure of hospitals. Specifically, we want to reduce the amount of time and number of people consumed by activities not central to patient care and service. Recall that less than 20 percent of current personnel time and cost is devoted to direct care. The categories targeted for attack are scheduling-coordinating, documentation, and ready-for-action time (structural idle time). Since the pilot approach adopted by the early implementers was not designed with the near-term goal of reducing overall cost, the new system at a minimum had to produce more time devoted to direct care and increased service (both in absolute terms and percentage of total effort). But even hospitals entering the process with near-term cost goals must take a step back and realize that the essence of restructuring (of almost any variety, in almost any industry) is rethinking where and how resources are deployed and consumed.

The results to date are right in line with expectations and imperatives. Those who have fully implemented protocols and documentation by exception have seen especially dramatic reductions in personnel time devoted to paperwork. In general, bedside nursing hours per patient and the percentage of nurses' time devoted to various aspects of direct care are up significantly. Typical results show that nurses are now devoting 45 to 50 percent of their time to direct care (as opposed to 35 to 40 percent before the restructuring). To avoid confusion with the earlier numbers, recall that the 16 percent of value added cited earlier for direct care was an average of all hospital employees. The nursing staff of course accounted for a disproportionate percentage of all direct care activities.

By and large, the improvement in bedside activities was "free." The changes were paid for by reductions in scheduling and coordinating and documentation. The most stunning reduction in documentation saw it decline from nearly 20 percent of the nursing staff's time to less than 5 percent. This is the true value of restructuring.

The model is not without its problems, however. In the old world, the nursing station was the center of all activities. Furthermore, it was a major congregation point. If you wanted to find a particular nurse, your best chance was to check with or call the nursing station. The new paradigm is much more decentralized. Bedside staff members are usually at the bedside; they do not just drop in from the nursing station to complete a given task or transaction. As a result, the units are much quieter places. As we look down the halls, we see only care givers as they move from patient to patient; they are not massed at the station. As good as this system is, it creates communication problems. Calling in to find a specific care giver can be frustrating; the odds are against finding that person at or near the nursing station. Some hospitals are experimenting with zone phones in the halls outside the block of rooms covered by a particular care team. This solution works reasonably well if the care teams' patients are clustered geographically and predictably. But this is not always the case or even possible. For the moment, intense team work is making do within these limitations, but a longer-term solution is needed. Perhaps further evolution of cellular technology will enable each care giver to carry a portable phone with direct access from outside callers (physicians, primarily). Sometime in the future, we may even see "robo-nurse," equipped with a small cellular headphone and carrying one or two other portable devices for data acquisition and simple blood tests. Until that day, a major opportunity awaits the telecommunications field to solve the new problems on patient-focused care centers.

Reviewing the value-added profile of the old and new models is all well and good, but it does not give a vivid picture of the true nature of the change that these hospitals have implemented. The experiences of one veteran nurse captures the change more dramatically and in human terms. She especially notices the differences on an extremely busy and stressful day. Now when things are really hectic, she goes home more physically tired than in the past. She has more things to do. But she does not go home and cry. That is what happened in the old world when the work load became overwhelming. She would just get frustrated—spending much of her day on the phone trying to get other people to do the things her patients needed. Eight hours of bickering, cajoling, screaming, and even stretching the truth when necessary were not rewarding. Now, even if she has to hurry between tasks, she and her partners can still get everything necessary done, and they have the discretion to defer things that are not critical. Best of all, the patients see and appreciate her efforts. This nurse probably does not know anything about value-added structures, but she is sure that neither she nor her patients would ever want to go back to the old ways.

Continuity of Care

Improving continuity of care was absolutely crucial to the success of the new model. Fortunately, progress toward this goal was relatively easy to make and to measure. The results have been dramatic along several dimensions.

The number of staff members interacting with a patient during a stay has been cut by more than 50 percent. The first hospital to implement the concepts of patient-focused care has seen the number fall from nearly sixty to fewer than twenty. Just think of all the separate individuals who have been eliminated from face-to-face contact with patient (phlebotomists, housekeepers, transporters, admitting staff, utilization review staff, and so forth).

In addition to developing multiskills, the other mechanism for enhancing continuity is to assure that the faces that the patient does see are consistent from day to day on the various shifts. This is a fairly straightforward issue for short-stay patients—especially those whose hospitalization is usually concentrated on weekdays (those having elective surgery, for example). Although it is harder to maintain continuity for longer-stay patients (such as medicine patients), we can still improve on today, when equal distribution of the work often receives a higher priority than continuity of care. In the future, we may see nurses working a period of, say, ten days on and ten days off to correspond to the expected stays of their patients. In general, the goal of continuity is made somewhat easier by the fact that the majority of patients on these units seldom need to leave the unit for services (from strangers). For example, on one surgical patient care center, more than 80 percent of the patients remain on the unit for their entire stay except for the trip to the operating room.

There is another dimension of continuity; that which occurs between physicians and care givers. At their best, patient-focused ideas can be applied to this relationship as well. With careful scheduling (of the useful kind), we have seen hospitals where a busy surgeon deals with just two care teams for all his or her patients over a ninety-day period. Less-active surgeons work with a broader variety of care teams, but we can usually meet the eighty-twenty rule; we can cater to the 20 percent of surgeons who provide 80 percent of demand. Even this set of priorities could be adjusted somewhat in a hospital that is seeking to use patient-focused care as a means of gaining market share. Surgeons who have been splitting their admissions between hospitals could, for example, be allocated a dedicated care team for a free ninety-day trial of patient-focused care—in exchange for bringing all their patients to the hospital during that period.

As time goes on, we will see the principles of continuity of care pushed to new levels and applied within specific functional areas. One hospital is contemplating major changes in the center handling prep, OR, and recovery room functions. Today this area is rife with narrow definitions of ownership. The patient is prepped and held for surgery by one staff person. During surgery, a circulating nurse coordinates and assists. After the procedure, the patient is recovered by another staff member. Although the patients may not be fully aware of these discontinuities, there can be major benefits to training employees to have all these skills and to assigning one professional to the patient throughout the entire process. Strange as it may seem, modeling this integrated process reveals that, with proper teaming, nurses could get more in-depth experience (measured as working with fewer

surgeons per year and doing more repetitions of the same procedures). Once instituted, the staffing levels would be no higher
than today's. The major stumbling block is the initial cross-training investment—primarily the training of prep nurses and circu-
lators to perform recovery tasks. Such innovations may need to
await changes in the educational system, so that the staff can be
prepared for this broader role through formal, rather than hospi-
tal-based, training.

Satisfaction

All the hospitals evaluated satisfaction in three areas: patients,
physicians, and staff. The results have been nearly uniformly
good, especially on the patient satisfaction dimension. There are
some limitations and caveats to note, however, before we review
some of the findings. First, each hospital used existing survey
instruments. This decision may seem logical (and it is) and necessary for a fair comparison, but it also presents some problems.
As we discussed in the very first chapter, hospitals and other
service businesses are not very adept at asking the right questions
of their customers. Almost all the ones used on existing question-
naires are asked in old-world terms (How was the admitting office?). In the future, patient-focused hospitals will need to develop
much more sophisticated tools to provide input to a CQI or TQM
process. Secondly, cross-institutional comparisons and bench-
marking are difficult because there was no one, standard questionnaire used at multiple sites. Third, we must remember that
these were very successful institutions to begin with; they already
enjoyed extremely high regard from their patients, doctors, and
employees. Showing improvement was therefore not necessarily
going to be an easy thing.

Findings indicated that patient satisfaction had made the
most uniform and dramatic improvements. Furthermore, these
were nearly immediate. One hospital that regularly used the
Press-Ganey organization to study patient perceptions discovered
that its medicine patient-focused care center went from being the

most poorly rated unit in the hospital to its best in the first month of operation. In addition, Press-Ganey stated that it was the largest one-month gain for a unit that it had recorded anywhere in the country. Areas that routinely improved significantly include responsiveness, the personal dimension of care, and the extent to which the patient felt informed about what was happening. One hospital even saw an improvement in patients' perceptions of the food, although it was the same as always. (Perhaps this reaction was due to the fact that a familiar face delivered it and picked it up). One hospital even told of overnight chemotherapy patients calling to schedule their next stay so they could be assured of getting on "the good unit."

Physician reaction was a bit more mixed. On the plus side, doctors were quite pleased with what they perceived as a higher level of patient care, greatly improved turnaround times for unit-based services, and improved (and more continuous) relationships with care givers. On the less positive side, changes in documentation procedures required that old habits be broken. The results along this dimension tended to be bimodal; the majority was reasonably satisfied with the new procedures, and the minority was vocal and very unhappy. Interestingly, the vocal-minority physicians tended not to be the most active admitters.

Staff satisfaction also improved, but there were some interesting twists. The most predictable improvement occurred in overall job satisfaction, sense of empowerment, positive feedback from patients, and appreciation of the reduced paperwork and process complexity. The areas that needed continuing attention mostly concerned communications; employees always want more, but the staff members on the new patient care centers seem to have insatiable appetites. Turnover (or even transfer) was astonishingly low on these units (of course, virtually all of the staff were volunteers and highly motivated). Eventually, these units will be staffed by more "average" employees, and management will need to discover new means of motivation if the momentum is to be maintained.

Even the most skeptical observer would be hard pressed

to find any evidence from the satisfaction surveys that would warrant a slowdown in the implementation of patient-focused care. But we are just at the beginning of a long process of transformation. More sophisticated measurements will be needed to assess these factors. We will also need new management tools that can address the problems and push the boundaries of performance even further.

Cost

No one has saved a nickel yet. But that statement does not really tell the whole story. The cost savings are still a bit downstream for the early (pilot) implementers. They knew this fact going into the process and feel they are on track. For the second wave of implementers, the savings are also downstream but much closer to the front end of the process (as previously stated, these are the hospitals that will be redesigning and redeploying selected bundles of services throughout their institutions over the next six to eighteen months). But even these observations do not tell the whole story of cost reduction and expectation.

Most of the early implementers modeled the economics of the new paradigm before beginning. By and large, those models anticipated cost savings on the order of 10 percent at the end of the process. In one case, after six months of its first pilot, one institution had an outside firm study the pilot and compare its operation to another unit in the hospital that cared for similar patients. The conclusion of the firm was that the new system was delivering care for 9 percent less than the traditional model. In general, these pioneering hospitals knew that the savings would only come when enough of the units had been restructured to permit the downsizing, consolidation, and (in some cases) elimination of central functions.

It is also becoming apparent that we have to reconsider how we compare costs. Because of changes in lengths of stay and ancillary consumption, the equation becomes a bit more complicated. One hospital found that gross revenue fell somewhat (due to shorter stays and fewer ancillaries) but that net revenue increased (because of dramatically reduced allowances and adjustments). This outcome, combined with expected declines in overall operating expenses, gives the CEO of that hospital great confidence in proceeding to full implementation.

Although no one has yet implemented patient-focused care using the housewide functional restructuring approach, the results of the models are intriguing and should produce results within six months of hospitalwide initiation. Several hospitals are committed to achieving a reduction of one FTE for every three FTEs that are restructured and redeployed. In other words, if there are currently 120 housekeepers, transporters, phlebotomists, couriers, and distribution staff members, it is likely that ninety will be redeployed and the remaining thirty laid off or eliminated through attrition. Even using a conservative estimate of $25,000 per FTE (salary and benefits), the result would be annual savings of $750,000—capable of repaying a typical investment in restructuring within one year of implementation.

Over the next two years or so, we should have much more definitive data on the economic performance of patient-focused care. By that time, some of the pioneering institutions will have completed their initial projects and restructured their central departments. In addition, perhaps a dozen more hospitals will have implemented at least the first wave of functional redeployment. We should expect continued good news and some surprises that may lead us to new insights about managing the patient-focused enterprise.

What Is Patient-Focused Care Like?

Perhaps the best way to conclude this chapter on results is to present another of our True-Life Adventures. This one focuses on an average morning for a patient—first in the old system and then in the patient-focused one. It is all too easy to lose sight of the human dimension of our business. These stories should serve to remind us of why we really go to work each day and may even inspire us to think about processes and work flows from the point of view of someone who does not feel very well to begin with: the patient.

"Good Morning, Mrs. Jones"

A disembodied voice intrudes in the darkness. "Mrs. Jones? Mrs. Jones?"

"Uh. What? What?" murmurs our semiconscious patient. "What time is it?"

"Good morning, Mrs. Jones. It's almost 6:00," the night nurse responds.

"In the morning? *What's wrong? Is there a fire? Did my heart stop?" asks Mrs. Jones, her annoyance gradually overcoming her sleepiness. "You just woke me up four hours ago to give me a sleeping tablet. What do you want now?"*

"Well, if you remember, your doctor ordered some tests for you last night, and we need to get started if they're going to be ready in time for her to see the results," the nurse tells her, with undertones of pride in this precisely orchestrated process.

"Yes, I do remember," Mrs. Jones replies. "But I also remember that she said she had several surgeries this morning at another hospital and wouldn't be here for rounds until at least 1:00. So what's the rush?"

I wish I could work in ICU, the nurse thinks wistfully. At least unconscious patients don't complain. "I don't make the rules, Mrs. Jones, and besides there are more than four hundred patients at this hospital, and we have lots and lots of tests to get done every day. This is the system that works for us," the nurse tells her patient.

"I guess I have no choice. What do I have to do?" asks Mrs. Jones.

"We need a urine sample, please. Here's the cup," responds the nurse, relieved that things were finally moving along.

"All right. I'll do that and then take a shower while I'm in the bathroom. At least I can be clean for the ordeal," Mrs. Jones responds.

"Well, normally *that would be just fine. But your doctor ordered some blood work, and the phlebotomist should be here any minute. So I'm afraid a shower is out of the question this morning,"* the nurse says, feeling a bit mean and beginning to understand why some patients get upset.

"Oh, very nice," says Mrs. Jones as sarcastically as possible.

Upon exiting the bathroom, an embarrassed Mrs. Jones hands the nurse her urine sample. "Where's this phlebotomist then?" she asks.

"I'm sure she'll be here soon. I'll take this sample to the collection point now. By the way, don't eat your breakfast until they've drawn the blood sample," orders the nurse as she leaves, obviously relieved to get out of the room and looking forward to ending her shift.

The minutes tick by. Seven o'clock and still no phlebotomist. Given the way the day began, Mrs. Jones is unsurprised when her breakfast tray is delivered. Her temper rises as the food cools on the overbed table. Still no phlebotomist. Out of the corner of her eye, she notices the housekeepers lurking—obviously wishing she would eat and get out of bed.

At last, the phlebotomist arrives. She is kind and reassuring as she expertly finds a vein and draws two tubes of blood. "Easy as you please, once they get to it." Mrs. Jones thinks.

Just as Mrs. Jones lifts the lid on her breakfast tray, a voice calls out, "Mrs. Jones, I'm Ted from transportation. I'll be taking you to radiology this morning."

"Now? I'm just starting breakfast," protests Mrs. Jones. "I know it's cold, but it's the only food I'll see for a while."

"Don't worry. I'll tell the ward clerk as we pass the nursing station to order you a late tray. When you get back to your room, you should have a hot breakfast waiting for you," Ted offers sympathetically. "We're in good shape for X ray. You're scheduled for 8:10 and it's now 7:45. Plenty of time to get you down there." Mrs. Jones puts on her robe and sits in the wheelchair. Ted hands her the chart to hold; it is already an impressively thick document, given that she has only been a patient for two days.

"Sorry about the elevators, Mrs. Jones," apologizes Ted as they arrive in X ray at 8:08. "I think they're planning to add elevators in next year's expansion project. I move twenty patients a day, and I always have to wait."

As Ted leaves, he gives her chart to the receptionist. Mrs. Jones sees that she is not alone. Eight other patients are waiting—some on gurneys, some in wheelchairs. I'm glad I'm here on time, she thinks. These patients must have been brought down early for their appointments. By 8:40, the naïveté of that initial assessment becomes apparent to her.

The technologist rescues Mrs. Jones at 8:45, and the chest film is done in no time. By 8:55, she and her chart are redeposited in the waiting area. It takes another twenty-five minutes for Mary (another transporter) to appear for the return trip. By 9:30 or so, she is back in her room—along with two housekeepers as it turns out. Although she is not thrilled, she realizes that they are nearly done. The fresh sheets and her soon-to-appear breakfast might put her in a better mood.

By 10:00, her patience is exhausted. She buzzes for the nurse. A few minutes later, the day-shift nurse appears. "Good morning, Mrs. Jones. What can I do for you?" she asks pleasantly.

"I'm waiting for my late breakfast tray. Has it arrived yet?" she inquires.

"No. But it shouldn't be much longer. When did you order it?" the nurse responds.

"Around 7:30, as I was being wheeled to X ray," answers Mrs. Jones.

"Let me make sure the day clerk got the order from the night clerk. I'm sure she did," the nurse offers.

"Can I get some coffee while we wait?" Mrs. Jones asks politely, not wanting to alienate this potential ally.

"Sure," the nurse answers. "I'll get someone to do that." And she disappears out the door.

Ten minutes later and no coffee. Mrs. Jones rings her call button. The day nurse appears in just a couple of minutes—without coffee. "What do you need, Mrs. Jones?" she asks, ever helpful.

"I was wondering about that coffee," comes the reply.

"You mean the aide hasn't been here yet? I'll go track him down right away. By the way, your breakfast tray should be here very soon," she says and disappears again.

"It might be faster just to track down the coffee yourself," Mrs. Jones mutters under her breath.

At 10:40, an aide appears in her room with coffee at the same time as a dietary employee walks in with her tray—complete with a mug of coffee. It never rains but it pours, she muses.

A bit worse for the early rising, poking, waiting, and harassment, she begins her breakfast. It is hot; she is ravenous. Life is sometimes good, even for prisoners.

As the first forkful of hash browns nears her mouth, a voice intrudes from the doorway. "Mrs. Jones, I'm Alice from EKG. Is now a good time?"

"Do I have a choice?" asks Mrs. Jones sarcastically.

"Well, I'm pretty booked up this morning, and you're my only patient on this floor. Your doctor wanted this done today," Alice answers, hoping that she has made her point politely.

"Very well, then. But let's be quick," snaps Mrs. Jones.

The EKG is mercifully brief. Mrs. Jones's hunger lets her ignore the unpleasant tepidness of her eggs as she resumes her breakfast. When she finishes, her next thought is of having a hot shower.

While enjoying the privacy and the steamy warmth, her shower is interrupted by a knock on the door. "Mrs. Jones? Mrs. Jones? Has EKG been in to see you yet this morning?" comes the familiar voice of the day nurse.

"Yes!" she answers, her irritation finally showing. Doesn't anyone know what's going on around here? she wonders.

As Mrs. Jones emerges from the bathroom feeling somewhat refreshed, her spirit is crushed as she sees her luncheon tray delivered.

This True-Life Adventure illustrates most of the major problems today's operating approach poses for patients—with the exception of all the paperwork and repetitive questions from

various staff members. Let us now take a look at these same transactions in the more flexible environment of patient-focused care.

"It's Your Wake-Up Call, Mrs. Jones"

*"Mrs. Jones? Mrs. Jones? It's 7 A.M. You wanted to be awakened
then,"* the nurse says.

"Good morning, Carol. Thank you very much," Mrs. Jones
*manages to say as she gradually comes out of her sleep. She no-
tices in the room not only Carol, her regular day-shift nurse,
but also Greg, her care giver on nights. They have obviously just
concluded their shift-change review of her record and progress.*

*"Today should be a pretty easy one for you, Mrs. Jones.
Just a few tests and all the television you can stand,"* Carol offers.
*"Everything you'll need is right here on the unit, and there's no
great rush since your doctor isn't expected until this afternoon,"*
she adds as she completes the process of taking vital signs.

*"Good. I'm hoping to find out if I can go home tomorrow.
By the way, my son is visiting around 11:30 this morning. Can
we get everything I need sorted out by then?"* Mrs. Jones asks.

*"I don't see why not. Would you like your room cleaned
before he arrives?"* the nurse responds.

*"That would be very nice. Also, he may want to eat while
he's here. Can you arrange something?"*

*"No problem. Well then, your breakfast will be here soon.
I think you'll have time for a shower, all right? By the way, we
need a urine sample. Just leave it in the bathroom after your
shower, and I'll pick it up,"* Carol suggests, handing her a specimen jar.

*Just as she emerges from her shower, she sees that breakfast
is on its way in. "This may not be a hotel, but they come pretty
close,"* Mrs. Jones muses.

*As she finishes her breakfast and turns off the morning news
program, Carol and her team mate, Anne, enter the room. "Mrs.
Jones, I'll take you down the hall to the X ray room whenever
you're ready. While we're down there, Anne will see to your
room."*

"Good. I feel like taking a little walk anyway," she answers.

The X ray goes smoothly, and Mrs. Jones stops for a few minutes on her way back to confer with Jerry, the unit clerk. He handled all the paperwork when she was admitted, and she wants to make sure everything is taken care of with her insurance company. Jerry assures her that there are no problems and even gives her an estimate of the copayment portion that she should expect to be billed for.

Her room is spotless when she returns. Carol soon reappears to arrange with her the rest of her morning.

"Let's see; it's 10 A.M. We've got plenty of time to do your EKG and draw a bit of blood for the lab. Would it be all right if Anne stops by in a few minutes? She'll be done well before your son arrives," Carol prompts.

"Sure. I'm all set for his visit anyway, and the room looks great," she answers.

Anne arrives a few minutes later and is finished with the EKG and the blood draw in less than ten minutes. "You're all done for today. Relax and enjoy your son's visit. The doctor called and said she'd be here around 3 P.M. You could even grab a nap after lunch," Anne says as she rolls her equipment out of the room.

Mrs. Jones's son arrives shortly before noon, and her luncheon tray is not far behind. Just as she begins to eat, Ms. Anderson, the unit director, enters the room with another tray. "Don't let me interrupt, but I thought I would see how you're doing and deliver this guest tray for your son. Are you comfortable?" Ms. Anderson asks.

"Thank you very much. Everything is just fine."

The old world is not always so horrible, and the patient-focused world will not always be so wonderful. But these stories contain much truth—truth about how we think about our hospitals' operations today and about how that thinking must change. We will have made remarkable progress if we simply begin to *notice* the problems our traditional model creates. That is the first step. The second and perhaps more difficult one is to begin to believe that we can *solve* those problems.

Epilogue:

The Patient-Focused

Enterprise

Understanding why we need patient-focused care and what it consists of is critical to moving forward with major change. This book has focused on these issues almost exclusively. But there is more. Questions of implementation will quickly come to the fore—issues of process, change management, culture change, detailed job design, and training. Hospitals today are facing these issues and beginning to answer the questions; their experience will eventually make it easier for other institutions to implement patient-focused care.

The second extension of patient-focused care involves the transformation of hospitals and systems into patient-focused enterprises. Whatever we may think of the various proposals and probable directions of health care reform, there is little doubt that the system has broken down. It is equally clear that much of what has made the system malfunction is being addressed by patient-focused care. The structural dimension is the crucial issue for the national health care system, just as it is for hospital operations.

The system is hopelessly fragmented. There are more than 400,000 physician "companies" (groups or individuals), six thousand hospitals, and a dizzying array of home health providers, clinics, diagnostic centers, surgery centers, long-term care facilities, and other sites and formats. Further, these figures do not include pharmacies, optical services, and dental and allied health professionals who hang out their own shingles. It should therefore not be surprising that insurance companies and other agencies have stepped into this mess to try to bring some order. In the process, they have added their own complexities to the system, so that providers must deal with hundreds of such agents offering thousands of plans and benefit packages.

At the same time, a patient's expectations of the system are almost pathetically naive. Although the members of some HMOs receive nearly coherent services, most patients would find that their most basic ideas about the system are false. The average patient might expect the various parts of the system to be well informed about his or her condition and progress, to be working in concert for the best outcome, and to be aware of the costs and benefits of various treatment options. Although one of these statements might be true for any given transaction, the probability of an overarching view of the situation is very small.

The frictional losses of such a system are colossal—that is, we put more into the system than we get out—even before we take into account the critical information that is either lost or duplicated as the transactions move inexorably forward. But there are no simple solutions. Proposals for a one-payer system will solve few if any of our information and cost problems. Such approaches purport to be capable of stripping away as much as 15 percent of total costs by the mere expedient of creating, in essence, just one bill for all payers. The cost problem involved in this dimension, though, is not the final package of software in hospital computers that produces either one kind of bill or two hundred kinds. The problem is the structure that insists on gathering all the data in the first place. It is unlikely that hospitals would stop gathering detailed charge data simply because only one type of bill was necessary. Hospitals are insatiable for the same kind of information to power the productivity measurement engine. Until the structure—and that mindset—changes, improving the final billing process will have little impact.

In the final analysis, the fundamental problems with the system boil down to two complex issues: public expectations and the incentive structure for providers. The first problem is likely to require generations to solve. Patients expect medicine and technology to fix nearly everything, and this expectation is aided and abetted by physicians' training. These two factors combine to contribute to make litigation the preferred means for bringing reality into line with expectation. When doctors are expected to do everything possible (and their training reinforces this), we should not be surprised to find disproportionate sums spent on the last few months of (often) low quality of life. Looking over every doctor's shoulder is not only the patient and the family but also a lawyer. This is not to say that there is not genuine malpractice; there is. But the entire culture must change if we are to bring any rationality to this dimension of the demand curve. Structural change will not be enough.

The other dimension of the problem can be addressed structurally, and in most cases this is what so-called health-care reform is all about. With minor exceptions, the only way now for providers to increase their wealth is to send out more bills. This situation is what must change. Hospital discounting will not help. Absent the full economic participation of doctors, this is little more than a cost-shifting and charge-unbundling game. If you doubt this, go to a city of your choice; listen to the hospitals complain about deep discounts; listen to selected employers crow about the deals they negotiated; and then look at total net revenues at all hospitals in the area. You can be virtually guaranteed to find that total net revenues are up. Furthermore, you will find that the number of physicians in the area is also up—and it is unlikely that as a group they are getting poorer. So who is winning this game? No one. And in the long run, this basis of competition is unsustainable; sooner or later, the people paying the bills will figure it out. It may take some time, though, since the shifting of costs is unlikely to stop until the hospital's last charge-paying patient receives a bill for $150 million for an appendectomy.

Whether we choose to approach these problems from the market side of the political spectrum or the mandate side, the structural features of the solution are likely to be rather similar. Whether the result is medical service companies or accountable health partnerships (in addition to more or less traditional HMOs), the competitive landscape will change forever. Once the basis of competiton truly shifts to at-risk (and probably capitated) arrangements, providers will need to assemble the current fragments into a coherent whole that is fully accountable to its customers. Wealth will be accumulated not by sending out more bills but by delivering effective care over the long run. The enterprise must be seamless and low cost. The best organizations will measure their success not just in financial terms but also by their customers' health status and reenrollment rates.

What do these policy issues have to do with patient-focused care? It can (and probably should) be elevated to the system or enterprise level as the basis of competition changes. It may need to be renamed in the process, but we should increasingly view patient-focused care as a paradigm that defines more than an operating approach. It is in a very real sense a change in our view of how health care organizations add value. Health care enterprises will need to justify their existence and actions by answering the question: how does this decision add value for the customer at the bedside, in the clinic, and at home? This is the question that our journey through patient-focused care brings us back to time and time again. Just as we should ask, "How does rolling a patient all through the hospital add value to a chest X ray?", so too we should begin to demand, "How do centralized corporate services add measurable value to patients and other customers?" Furthermore, the sites and formats of care in the enterprise of the future will go far beyond the inpatient setting and the emergency room. Physician offices, home care services, and even long-term care become additional components to be assembled and restructured. Patient-focused care concepts should be brought to bear on this process if we are to avoid merely reassembling today's suboptimal pieces and hoping that things work out.

This is a great challenge, because changes in format do not guarantee changes in structure. Great opportunities are missed—or at best deferred. As an example, think about a hospital that is owned and operated by an HMO, and all of the patients are its own plan members. Such hospitals exist today. If you were to walk through such a hospital, you would be unlikely to suspect that it was any different from a similar, non-HMO facility. Its operating structure, design, and layout would seem quite familiar. You would walk in the front door and see an admitting office. But what purpose does it fulfill? Exaggerating a bit, there are no strangers admitted to the hospital, patients' costs are almost all covered by the plan, and the doctor who referred the patient is probably employed by the HMO. Why not just have an electronic card reader that refers the patient to an assigned bed? The success that was enabled by the change in format (HMO versus traditional) probably masked the opportunity to push the gains even further and truly change the industry. It is this sort of opportunity that we should challenge ourselves to find as our field undergoes reform in the years ahead.

The next few years will be exciting and challenging. This period will see the first hospitals to complete their restructuring. It will also witness scores of other hospitals entering the process. Ambulatory care services will be incorporated into the model, and the first patient-focused outpatient centers will appear. Early adapters will use patient-focused care to increase their market shares and attract managed-care customers by offering superior service at competitive or below-market prices.

Patient-focused care will emerge as the dominant operational paradigm for hospitals over the remainder of the decade. As this process occurs, we can expect changes in the supportive infrastructure of the system. We may see nurses and allied health professionals trained more broadly before they enter the work force. We can hope to see regulation brought into line with technological change and our new view of patient care operations. At the same time, there will be dislocations as well. Some of our employees will not make the journey with us—either because there is no room for them or because their values are not consistent with the goals of patient-focused care. This situation is sad but true, and we should proceed with our eyes open.

When will we be done? Never. We will have failed in part of our mission if patient-focused care is seen as the destination—one "thing" to be accomplished. We must recognize that we are on a journey and that further progress and renewal are part of it. Continuous improvement must be our goal. If it is not, we will only have succeeded in creating the next edifice that must be razed by future generations. We can do better.

Recommended

Readings

Anderson, H. J. "New Planning Models." *Hospitals*, Feb. 5, 1993, pp. 20–22.

Booz·Allen & Hamilton. "Operations Strategy—The Missing Ingredient." Chicago: Booz·Allen & Hamilton, 1988.

Booz·Allen & Hamilton. "Operational Restructuring—The 'Patient-Focused' Hospital." Chicago: Booz·Allen & Hamilton, 1990.

Booz·Allen & Hamilton. "The Patient-Focused Hospital: Facility and Cost Implications." Chicago: Booz·Allen & Hamilton, 1990.

Brider, P. "The Move to Patient-Focused Care." *American Journal of Nursing*, Sept. 1992, pp. 26–33.

Cassidy, J. "Patient-Focused Delivery Promises to Reshape Hospitals." *Health Progress*, May 1992, pp. 20–21.

Crichton, M. "A Revolution in Patient Care." *Vanderbilt Medicine*, internal publication of Vanderbilt University, Spring 1990, pp. 19–23.

Health Care Advisory Board. *Hospital of the Future*. Vol. 1: *Toward a Twenty-First Century Hospital—Redesigning Patient Care.* Washington, D. C.: Health Care Advisory Board, 1992.

Jacobsen, J. T. "Better Planning Needed to Strengthen Patient Care Systems." *Computers in Healthcare,* Oct. 1992, pp. 30–32.

Lathrop, J. P. "The Patient-Focused Hospital." *Healthcare Forum Journal,* Jul.–Aug. 1991, pp. 16–21.

Lathrop, J. P. "The Odyssey." *Healthcare Forum Journal,* Nov.–Dec. 1992, pp. 76–78.

Lathrop, J. P. "The Patient-Focused Hospital." *Healthcare Forum Journal,* May–June 1992, pp. 76–78.

Lathrop, J. P. "The Patient-Focused Hospital—A Patient Care Concept." *Journal of the Society for Health Systems,* 1992, *3*(2), 33–50.

Lathrop, J. P. "The Do-It-Yourself Restructuring Test." *Healthcare Forum Journal,* May–June 1993, pp. 108–111.

Lumsdon, K. "Form Follows Function." *Hospitals,* Feb. 5, 1993, pp. 22–26.

McQueen, H. E., Jr. "The Healthcare CIO's Role in Business Process Redesign." *Computers in Healthcare,* Feb. 1993, pp. 24–26.

"Model for the New Millenium." *Hospital Development,* Sept. 1992, p. 5.

"Operational Restructuring—Nineteen Pioneering Models." *Healthcare Forum Journal,* Jul.–Aug. 1992, pp. 43–61.

Peters, T. *Liberation Management.* New York: Knopf, 1992.

Scahill, M. "Care 2000 Program Refocuses on Patients at Mercy in San Diego." *Computers in Healthcare,* Oct. 1992, pp. 30–32.

Sherer, J. L. "Changing Cultures." *Hospitals,* Feb. 5, 1993, pp. 18–19.

Sherer, J. L. "Putting Patients First." *Hospitals,* Feb. 5, 1993, pp. 14–18.

Siler, J. F. "Hospital, Heal Thyself." *Business Week,* Aug. 27, 1990.

Smith, J. "The Patient-Focused Hospital." *Hospital Management International,* 1990, pp. 33–50.

Soviee, M. "Redesigning Our Future: Whose Responsibility Is It?" *Nursing Economics*, Jan.–Feb. 1990, *8*(1).

"A Taste of Things to Come." *Hospital Development*, Nov. 1990.

Weber, D. Q. "Six Models of Patient-Focused Care." *Healthcare Forum Journal*, Jul.–Aug. 1991.